Sex Differences in Brain Disorders
Emerging Transcriptomic Evidence

PROCEEDINGS OF A WORKSHOP

Lisa Bain, Sheena M. Posey Norris, and Clare Stroud, *Rapporteurs*

Forum on Neuroscience and Nervous System Disorders

Board on Health Sciences Policy

Health and Medicine Division

The National Academies of
SCIENCES • ENGINEERING • MEDICINE

THE NATIONAL ACADEMIES PRESS
Washington, DC
www.nap.edu

THE NATIONAL ACADEMIES PRESS   500 Fifth Street, NW   Washington, DC 20001

This activity was supported by contracts between the National Academy of Sciences and Alzheimer's Association; Cohen Veterans Bioscience; Department of Health and Human Services' Food and Drug Administration (5R13FD005362-05 and 1R13FD005362-06) and National Institutes of Health (NIH) (75N98019F00469 [Under Master Base HHSN263201800029I]) through the National Center for Complementary and Integrative Health, National Eye Institute, National Institute of Environmental Health Sciences, National Institute of Mental Health, National Institute of Neurological Disorders and Stroke, National Institute on Aging, National Institute on Alcohol Abuse and Alcoholism, National Institute on Drug Abuse, NIH Blueprint for Neuroscience Research, and NIH BRAIN Initiative; Department of Veterans Affairs (36C24E20C0009); Eisai Inc.; Eli Lilly and Company; Foundation for the National Institutes of Health; Gatsby Charitable Foundation; Janssen Research & Development, LLC; Lundbeck Research USA; Merck Research Laboratories; The Michael J. Fox Foundation for Parkinson's Research; National Multiple Sclerosis Society; National Science Foundation (DBI-1839274); One Mind; Sanofi; Society for Neuroscience; Takeda Pharmaceuticals International, Inc.; and Wellcome Trust. Any opinions, findings, conclusions, or recommendations expressed in this publication do not necessarily reflect the views of any organization or agency that provided support for the project.

International Standard Book Number-13: 978-0-309-26510-2
International Standard Book Number-10: 0-309-26510-X
Digital Object Identifier: https://doi.org/10.17226/26058

Additional copies of this publication are available from the National Academies Press, 500 Fifth Street, NW, Keck 360, Washington, DC 20001; (800) 624-6242 or (202) 334-3313; http://www.nap.edu.

Copyright 2021 by the National Academy of Sciences. All rights reserved.

Printed in the United States of America

Suggested citation: National Academies of Sciences, Engineering, and Medicine. 2021. *Sex differences in brain disorders: Emerging transcriptomic evidence: Proceedings of a workshop*. Washington, DC: The National Academies Press. https://doi.org/10.17226/26058.

The National Academies of
SCIENCES · ENGINEERING · MEDICINE

The **National Academy of Sciences** was established in 1863 by an Act of Congress, signed by President Lincoln, as a private, nongovernmental institution to advise the nation on issues related to science and technology. Members are elected by their peers for outstanding contributions to research. Dr. Marcia McNutt is president.

The **National Academy of Engineering** was established in 1964 under the charter of the National Academy of Sciences to bring the practices of engineering to advising the nation. Members are elected by their peers for extraordinary contributions to engineering. Dr. John L. Anderson is president.

The **National Academy of Medicine** (formerly the Institute of Medicine) was established in 1970 under the charter of the National Academy of Sciences to advise the nation on medical and health issues. Members are elected by their peers for distinguished contributions to medicine and health. Dr. Victor J. Dzau is president.

The three Academies work together as the **National Academies of Sciences, Engineering, and Medicine** to provide independent, objective analysis and advice to the nation and conduct other activities to solve complex problems and inform public policy decisions. The National Academies also encourage education and research, recognize outstanding contributions to knowledge, and increase public understanding in matters of science, engineering, and medicine.

Learn more about the National Academies of Sciences, Engineering, and Medicine at **www.nationalacademies.org**.

The National Academies of
SCIENCES · ENGINEERING · MEDICINE

Consensus Study Reports published by the National Academies of Sciences, Engineering, and Medicine document the evidence-based consensus on the study's statement of task by an authoring committee of experts. Reports typically include findings, conclusions, and recommendations based on information gathered by the committee and the committee's deliberations. Each report has been subjected to a rigorous and independent peer-review process and it represents the position of the National Academies on the statement of task.

Proceedings published by the National Academies of Sciences, Engineering, and Medicine chronicle the presentations and discussions at a workshop, symposium, or other event convened by the National Academies. The statements and opinions contained in proceedings are those of the participants and are not endorsed by other participants, the planning committee, or the National Academies.

For information about other products and activities of the National Academies, please visit www.nationalacademies.org/about/whatwedo.

PLANNING COMMITTEE ON SEX DIFFERENCES IN BRAIN DISORDERS[1]

ERIC NESTLER (*Chair*), Icahn School of Medicine at Mount Sinai
LI GAN, Weill Cornell Medical College
JOHN KRYSTAL, Yale University
HEATHER SNYDER, Alzheimer's Association
RITA VALENTINO, National Institute on Drug Abuse
DONNA WERLING, University of Wisconsin–Madison
STEVIN ZORN, MindImmune Therapeutics, Inc.

Health and Medicine Division Staff

CLARE STROUD, Director, Forum on Neuroscience and Nervous System Disorders
SHEENA M. POSEY NORRIS, Program Officer
PHOENIX WILSON, Senior Program Assistant (*until October 2020*)
ANDREW M. POPE, Senior Director, Board on Health Sciences Policy

---

[1] The National Academies of Sciences, Engineering, and Medicine's planning committees are solely responsible for organizing the workshop, identifying topics, and choosing speakers. The responsibility for the published Proceedings of a Workshop rests with the workshop rapporteurs and the institution.

FORUM ON NEUROSCIENCE AND NERVOUS SYSTEM DISORDERS[1]

FRANCES JENSEN (*Co-Chair*), University of Pennsylvania
JOHN KRYSTAL (*Co-Chair*), Yale University
SUSAN AMARA, National Institute of Mental Health
RITA BALICE-GORDON, Muna Therapeutics
KATJA BROSE, Chan Zuckerberg Initiative
EMERY BROWN, Harvard Medical School and Massachusetts Institute of Technology
JOSEPH BUXBAUM, Icahn School of Medicine at Mount Sinai
SARAH CADDICK, Gatsby Charitable Foundation
MARIA CARRILLO, Alzheimer's Association
EDWARD CHANG, University of California, San Francisco
TIMOTHY COETZEE, National Multiple Sclerosis Society
JONATHAN COHEN, Princeton University
ROBERT CONLEY, Eli Lilly and Company
JAMES DESHLER, National Science Foundation
BILLY DUNN, Food and Drug Administration
MICHAEL EGAN, Merck Research Laboratories
NITA FARAHANY, Duke University
JOSHUA GORDON, National Institute of Mental Health
MAGALI HAAS, Cohen Veterans Bioscience
RAMONA HICKS, One Mind
RICHARD HODES, National Institute on Aging
STUART HOFFMAN, Department of Veterans Affairs
JONATHAN HORSFORD, National Institute of Dental and Craniofacial Research
YASMIN HURD, Icahn School of Medicine at Mount Sinai
STEVEN HYMAN, Broad Institute of Massachusetts Institute of Technology and Harvard University
MICHAEL IRIZARRY, Eisai Inc.
GEORGE KOOB, National Institute on Alcohol Abuse and Alcoholism
WALTER KOROSHETZ, National Institute of Neurological Disorders and Stroke
STORY LANDIS, National Institute of Neurological Disorders and Stroke
ALAN LESHNER, American Association for the Advancement of Science (Emeritus)
JOSEPH MENETSKI, Foundation for the National Institutes of Health

---

[1] The National Academies of Sciences, Engineering, and Medicine's forums and roundtables do not issue, review, or approve individual documents. The responsibility for the published Proceedings of a Workshop rests with the workshop rapporteurs and the institution.

JOHN NGAI, National Institutes of Health BRAIN Initiative
STEVEN PAUL, Karuna Therapeutics, Inc.
SARAH SHEIKH, Takeda Pharmaceuticals International, Inc.
TODD SHERER, The Michael J. Fox Foundation for Parkinson's Research
DAVID SHURTLEFF, National Center for Complementary and Integrative Health
SANTA TUMMINIA, National Eye Institute
NORA VOLKOW, National Institute on Drug Abuse
ANDREW WELCHMAN, Wellcome Trust
DOUG WILLIAMSON, Lundbeck
RICHARD WOYCHIK, National Institute of Environmental Health Sciences
STEVIN ZORN, MindImmune Therapeutics, Inc.

Health and Medicine Division Staff

CLARE STROUD, Forum Director
CHANEL MATNEY, Program Officer (*from October 2020*)
SHEENA M. POSEY NORRIS, Program Officer
PHOENIX WILSON, Senior Program Assistant (*until October 2020*)
KIMBERLY SUTTON, Senior Program Assistant (*from October 2020*)
CHRISTIE BELL, Finance Business Partner (*from October 2020*)
BARDIA MASSOUDKHAN, Senior Finance Business Partner (*until September 2020*)
ANDREW M. POPE, Senior Director, Board on Health Sciences Policy

Reviewers

This Proceedings of a Workshop was reviewed in draft form by individuals chosen for their diverse perspectives and technical expertise. The purpose of this independent review is to provide candid and critical comments that will assist the National Academies of Sciences, Engineering, and Medicine in making each published proceedings as sound as possible and to ensure that it meets the institutional standards for quality, objectivity, evidence, and responsiveness to the charge. The review comments and draft manuscript remain confidential to protect the integrity of the process.

We thank the following individuals for their review of this proceedings:

JANINE CLAYTON, National Institutes of Health
DAVID PAGE, Massachussetts Institute of Technology
THEODORE PRICE, The University of Texas at Dallas
MARIANNE SENEY, University of Pittsburgh

Although the reviewers listed above provided many constructive comments and suggestions, they were not asked to endorse the content of the proceedings nor did they see the final draft before its release. The review of this proceedings was overseen by **ELI ADASHI,** Brown University. He was responsible for making certain that an independent examination of this proceedings was carried out in accordance with standards of the National Academies and that all review comments were carefully considered. Responsibility for the final content rests entirely with the rapporteurs and the National Academies.

Contents

1   INTRODUCTION AND BACKGROUND   1
    Workshop Objectives, 2
    Organization of the Proceedings, 4

2   TRANSCRIPTOMIC EVIDENCE FOR SEX DIFFERENCES
    IN STRESS- AND REWARD-RELATED DISORDERS   5
    Depression, 6
    Posttraumatic Stress Disorder, 8
    Addiction, 10
    Pain, 11
    Additional Factors Contributing to Sex Differences in Stress-
       and Reward-Related Disorders, 13

3   TRANSCRIPTOMIC EVIDENCE FOR SEX DIFFERENCES IN
    NEURODEVELOPMENTAL AND NEURODEGENERATIVE
    DISORDERS   15
    Autism, 16
    Schizophrenia, 19
    Alzheimer's Disease, 21
    Tauopathies, 24

4   MOVING FORWARD   29
    Technological Innovation to Drive Progress, 30
    Accounting for Sex Differences in Therapeutic Development, 33

Policy Implications of Incorporating Sex as a Biological Variable
  into Research and Drug Development, 34
Additional Areas for Future Research, 39
Closing Thoughts, 40

APPENDIXES

A References   41
B Workshop Agenda   47

1

Introduction and Background[1]

Accumulating evidence gathered over the past three decades has demonstrated a biological basis for differences between men and women with respect to clinical features and treatment responses to several neuropsychiatric, neurodevelopmental, and neurodegenerative disorders. Dramatic sex differences have also been identified in the brain transcriptomes of individuals with multiple brain disorders, including depression, posttraumatic stress disorder, and autism. The brain transcriptome includes all of the messenger RNA as well as the non-protein-coding RNA molecules expressed in brain tissue and thus represents gene activity. To explore these sex-based transcriptomic differences further, the National Academies of Sciences, Engineering, and Medicine's (the National Academies') Forum on Neuroscience and Nervous System Disorders (Neuroscience Forum) hosted a workshop on September 23, 2020, titled Sex Differences in Brain Disorders: Emerging Transcriptomic Evidence and Implications for Therapeutic Development. The workshop brought together a broad spectrum of stakeholders to share cutting-edge emerging evidence, discuss challenges, and identify future opportunities and potential directions.

This workshop explored the evolving understanding of sex differences in brain disorders, as reflected in previous reports and workshops convened

---

[1] The planning committee's role was limited to planning the workshop, and the Proceedings of a Workshop was prepared by the workshop rapporteurs as a factual summary of what occurred at the workshop. Statements, recommendations, and opinions expressed are those of individual presenters and participants, and have not been endorsed or verified by the National Academies of Sciences, Engineering, and Medicine. They should not be construed as reflecting any group consensus.

by the National Academies. Two decades ago, an Institute of Medicine (IOM) report asked whether sex matters in explorations of the biological contributions to human health. In that report, Mary-Lou Pardue, chair of the IOM Committee on Understanding the Biology of Sex and Gender Differences answered, "Sex does matter. It matters in ways that we did not expect. Undoubtedly, it also matters in ways that we have not begun to imagine" (IOM, 2001).

Ten years after that report, the Neuroscience Forum hosted a workshop on Sex Differences and Implications for Translational Neuroscience Research (IOM, 2011). By then, understanding of sex differences at the biological level had advanced considerably. Yet, in the summary from the 2010 workshop, Vivian Pinn, then the director of the Office of Research on Women's Health at the National Institutes of Health (NIH), noted that sex-specific research had been stymied by a limited focus on clinical studies. Molecular- and cellular-level research, she said, was essential to understanding sex differences in health.

Now, 10 years after the 2010 workshop and 20 years after the 2000 IOM report, recent advances in developing tools and technologies for molecular- and cellular-level research have fueled further advances and investigators are vigorously pursuing this research, said Rita Valentino, director of the Division of Neuroscience and Behavior at the National Institute on Drug Abuse.

The increased focus on sex differences has emerged in part as a result of a 2016 NIH mandate requiring that all NIH-funded research consider sex as a biological variable, said workshop chair Eric Nestler, Nash Family Professor of Neuroscience at the Icahn School of Medicine at Mount Sinai. Nestler called this mandate "transformational." For many years, his lab, like many others, had studied male rodents only, reasoning that including females would require twice or more as many animals and add too much complexity. In recent years, however, he and many other scientists have discovered striking sex differences across the spectrum of nervous system phenomena in both health and disease. Moreover, recent molecular approaches have revealed differences at the transcriptomic level between men and women with certain neurological or psychiatric disorders in human postmortem brains as well as between males and females in animal models of these disorders, said Nestler. The results of Nestler's and other scientists' studies suggest that some brain disorders in men and women, despite being similar with respect to behavioral presentations, may have dramatically different underlying biology.

WORKSHOP OBJECTIVES

The workshop was designed to explore emerging data about sex differences in the underlying biology of many different brain disorders with a focus on transcriptomic evidence; to consider how this evidence may advance understanding of brain disorder pathophysiology; to examine potential opportunities for applying this knowledge in the development of improved sex-specific treatments; and to review obstacles that must be overcome to realize this potential (see Box 1-1). Nestler noted that studying the impact of sex in a binary way—male and female—excludes people who do not fall along the male/female binary, for example, transgender individuals, those who have transitioned sex, and intersex individuals. Although this area of research is extremely important, he said, it is difficult to study in animal models, and the lack of availability of human brain tissue from nonbinary individuals makes human studies equally challenging.

Research presented at the workshop by individual participants is not a systematic review of the scientific landscape, but rather examples of emerging transcriptomic evidence for sex differences in brain disorders. Due to time restrictions, this 1-day workshop also did not include a robust discussion on other important issues such as a framework for approaching sex

---

BOX 1-1
Statement of Task

This public workshop will bring together experts and key stakeholders from academia, government, industry, and nonprofit organizations to explore emerging evidence regarding differences in transcriptomic abnormalities that occur in the brains of men versus women with a variety of brain disorders including depression, posttraumatic stress disorder, drug addiction, neurodegenerative conditions, and other brain disorders.

Invited presentations and discussions will be designed to:

- Review the landscape of emerging evidence regarding sex differences in transcriptomic abnormalities in a variety of brain disorders and discuss how this can be used to advance understanding of brain disorder pathophysiology.
- Explore ramifications for therapeutic development for these disorders, including identification of new targets, implications for preclinical and clinical study design, regulatory considerations, and potential sex-specific treatments.
- Discuss open research questions and opportunities to move the field forward.

The committee will develop the agenda for the workshop, select and invite speakers and discussants, and moderate the discussions. A proceedings of the presentations and discussions at the workshop will be prepared by a designated rapporteur in accordance with institutional guidelines.

differences in health and disease, or the merits and limitations of comparative studies apart from those in humans and mice, due to time restrictions.

ORGANIZATION OF THE PROCEEDINGS

The workshop was organized around several psychiatric and neurological disorders with evidence of biological differences according to sex. Chapter 2 focuses on stress- and reward-related disorders; Chapter 3 explores neurodevelopmental and neurodegenerative disorders. Chapter 4 transitions to a focus on policy implications and how federal agencies, industry, and nonprofit organizations can partner to leverage this new biology of sex differences to improve diagnostics and therapeutics for a range of brain disorders.

2

Transcriptomic Evidence for Sex Differences in Stress- and Reward-Related Disorders

HIGHLIGHTS

- Stress-related disorders show a robust sex bias, which is reflected in transcriptional profiles (Valentino).
- Non-genomic mechanisms, including environmental exposures, hormones, and societal pressures, may also drive sex differences in brain disorders (Lubin, Nestler, Seney).
- Transcriptome analyses in post-mortem brain tissue have demonstrated highly distinct profiles and gene networks with little overlap between men and women with depression, and these findings have been replicated in mouse models (Issler, Seney).
- Genomic and transcriptomic differences seen in posttraumatic stress disorder implicate different immune and interneuron pathways in males and females (Girgenti).
- Mouse studies suggest that adolescent stress drives sex differences in preference for cocaine, which are reflected in transcriptional differences (Walker).
- Transcriptomic studies indicate that sex differences in the peripheral immune system contribute to the transition from acute to chronic pain (Price).
- Sex-specific transcriptomic differences may translate into different therapeutic targets for men and women with chronic pain and other stress-related disorders (Price).

> NOTE: These points were made by the individual speakers identified above; they are not intended to reflect a consensus among workshop participants.

Stress-related disorders show a very robust sex bias, and thus provide a model for elucidating how sex differences at a molecular level translate to sex differences in expression and prevalence of a disease, said Rita Valentino. For example, major depressive disorder (MDD), anxiety, post-traumatic stress disorder (PTSD), and chronic pain disorders are nearly twice as prevalent in females as in males. Even substance use disorders, which are more prevalent in males but have shown increasing prevalence in females, appear to be linked to stress in females, said Valentino. She added that females with substance use disorders demonstrate a higher propensity for stress-induced relapse and a higher incidence of comorbid stress-related psychiatric disorders.

Valentino added that cognitive and affective features associated with depression, anxiety, PTSD, and pain disorders—negative affect, increased arousal, and reward deficit—are also linked to stress in that they have a common circuitry that interacts with stress circuitry. Comparing sex differences in transcriptional profiles across these disorders may provide clues about what governs the differential expression of symptoms, she said.

DEPRESSION

MDD affects approximately 19 million Americans each year (Kessler et al., 2003). The paucity of effective pharmacological treatments for depression may result from the heterogeneity of the disease, including sex differences, said Marianne Seney, assistant professor in the translational neuroscience program in the Department of Psychiatry at the University of Pittsburgh. She noted that compared with men, women are approximately twice as likely to have a single episode of depression and four times as likely to have recurrent depression. Women also have more symptoms, more severe symptoms, and higher subjective distress. In terms of comorbidities, depressed women have a higher incidence of comorbid anxiety disorders, while depressed men have a higher incidence of substance use disorders, said Seney.

The questions she and other scientists have set out to answer is whether these sex differences reflect the involvement of different biological pathways and/or sex-specific brain pathology, and whether a better understanding of these pathways and pathology may inform the future development of sex-specific treatments.

Seney suggested two different hypotheses regarding sex differences in the molecular pathology of depression. Men and women could have similar pathological changes moderated by sex-related factors such as gonadal hormones, or different pathologies altogether, she said. To explore these hypotheses, her lab and others have investigated gene-expression changes in brain circuits involved in mood regulation. They have used large-scale transcriptomic studies conducted using unbiased approaches such as microarray or RNA sequencing technologies.

For example, in what Seney called a tour-de-force study, Eric Nestler's lab used transcriptomic approaches to analyze a large cohort of well-characterized post-mortem brains across six different brain regions involved in mood regulation (Labonté et al., 2017). The results, she said, were striking: Across the cortical and subcortical brain regions they examined, they found that men and women with depression had distinct transcriptional profiles with very little overlap.

Next, they wanted to examine upstream drivers of these sex-specific differences. For this, they used an innovative technique called weighted gene co-expression network analysis (WGCNA) to identify gene modules (sets of genes whose expression is highly correlated across subjects). WGCNA enables investigators to identify gene networks with common functions and examine the commonalities and differences in expression modules between different populations (e.g., male versus female). This technique enabled Nestler and colleagues to identify sex-specific transcriptional networks in MDD. Within one female-specific module, they identified a candidate "hub" gene called *DUSP6*, which is highly connected to other genes in the network and differentially expressed in depressed women across all brain regions examined, said Seney. They went on to show in mouse models that reducing expression of *DUSP6* in the mouse prefrontal cortex drives stress susceptibility in female, but not male, mice.

Seney's lab replicated Nestler's work, demonstrating the same molecular changes using a different set of post-mortem brains. She said this confirmed that the sex-specific transcriptional alterations in MDD is a "real" phenomenon. Interestingly, of the small number of genes that were differentially expressed in both sexes, about 75 percent were changed in opposite directions in depressed men and women (Seney et al., 2018) (see Figure 2-1).

In total, Seney's lab showed that in more than 1,000 genes, there was a significant interaction of sex and disease, meaning that these 1,000 genes were altered differently in depressed men and women. She noted that only about 1 percent of those genes were differentially expressed in non-psychiatric control subjects. Moreover, mouse studies have suggested that

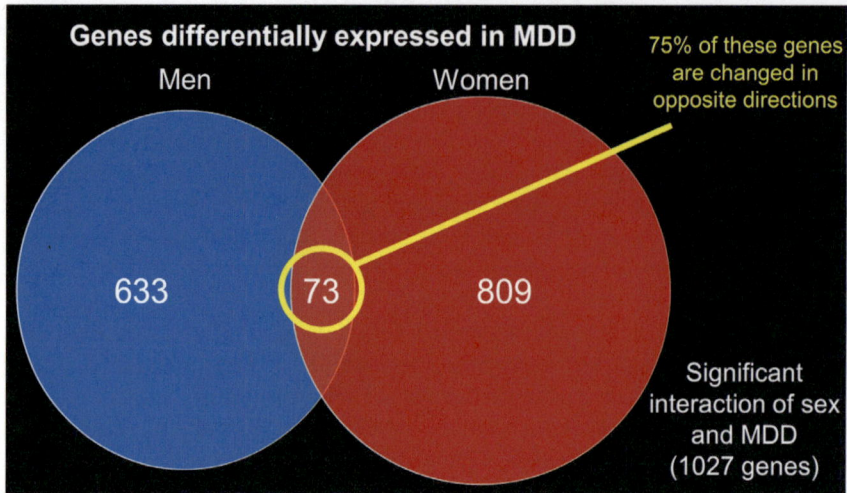

FIGURE 2-1 Distinct transcriptional changes in men and women with MDD.
NOTE: MDD = major depressive disorder.
SOURCES: Presented by Marianne Seney, September 23, 2020; adapted from Seney et al., 2018.

some of these sex differences are independent of hormone levels, she said. Her lab went on to show that differentially expressed genes were enriched for synapse structure, function, and organization (decreased expression in men versus increased expression in women) and immune function (increased expression or no change in men versus decreased expression in women). They also showed that depressed men have increased expression of microglia-specific genes (microglia being the resident immune cells of the brain) while depressed women have decreased expression.

Seney suggested that these studies have uncovered potential novel targets for the development of sex-specific depression treatments. They further suggest the possibility that treatments effective in men may be ineffective or even deleterious in women, and vice versa, she said.

POSTTRAUMATIC STRESS DISORDER

As with depression, sex-specific genomic and transcriptomic differences are seen in PTSD, said Matthew Girgenti, research scientist in psychiatry at the Yale School of Medicine. PTSD also has a high degree of comorbidity with depression, he said. Characterized by an uncontrollable and persistent state of fear triggered by a traumatic memory or event, PTSD is particularly prevalent among soldiers, with as many as 30 percent of returning soldiers found to have PTSD within 1 year of return from deployment, said Girgenti. The prevalence is much lower yet still substantial—about 8 percent—in the general population, according to the National Center for PTSD.[1] Given that PTSD is triggered by an outside environmental effect, it is a disorder for which epigenetics likely plays a key role, yet there are also heritable genetic components (Blacker et al., 2019). Moreover, genome-wide association studies (GWASs) with large diverse cohorts of PTSD cases and controls indicate that the heritability of PTSD is much higher in females than in males and nearly as high as schizophrenia in terms of heritability (Nievergelt et al., 2019). According to Girgenti, this means that about 10 percent of women will develop PTSD during their lifetime and are nearly twice as likely as men to develop PTSD after a traumatic event.

The neurobiology of PTSD has focused on regions of the brain that have been implicated in animal studies of fear—the prefrontal cortex, amygdala, and hippocampus (Nees et al., 2018). Girgenti's lab has conducted a large multi-omics project in post-mortem brain tissue, looking at four areas of the prefrontal cortex—the orbital frontal cortex, anterior cingulate, subgenual, and dorsolateral prefrontal cortex. These studies have shown that gene expression changes overwhelmingly occur in the orbital frontal cortex and dorsolateral prefrontal cortex, with genes involved in synaptic organization tending to be up-regulated, and genes related to glia and gliogenesis tending to be down-regulated, Girgenti said (Girgenti et al., 2021). He noted that this same phenomenon is seen in other neuropsychiatric disorders, including MDD.

Girgenti and colleagues examined the impact of multiple covariates on differential gene expression and found, to their surprise, that the overwhelming amount of differential variance was caused by sex. In females, substantial gene expression changes were seen in three brain regions, while in males, differential gene expression occurred only in one region, and there was very little overlap between male and female brains in terms of their gene expression profiles.

Using WGCNA, they determined that a gene module associated with female PTSD is enriched for markers of endothelial cells, while gene modules associated with male PTSD are enriched for markers of microglia and endothelial cells. Girgenti concluded that there is an overwhelming immune response resulting from the top sex-specific genes in both males and females, but that the genes and pathways differ between the sexes. Digging deeper, they conducted transcriptome-wide association studies (TWASs), which, in combination with GWAS, enabled the identification of one of the most highly significant female-specific, PTSD-associated modules (coral2) and the key driver of this module—a gene involved in interneuron synapse forma-

---

[1] To learn more, see https://www.ptsd.va.gov (accessed November 27, 2020).

tion called *ELFN1*. Girgenti suggested that *ELFN1* may confer significant genetic liability for PTSD, specifically in females.

The large number of gene expression changes suggested that there would likely be changes in cell-type proportions, said Girgenti. Using bulk sequencing RNA data combined with single-cell data, they demonstrated a significant increase in excitatory neurons and a decrease in astrocytes in females, and an increase in oligodendrocyte precursor cells and endothelial cells in males.

Girgenti and colleagues have also used their transcriptomic data to conduct drug repositioning analyses, a technique that predicts which drugs on the market might target the genes identified as being involved in a particular disorder. This analysis suggested that another gene they linked to PTSD—*PLEKHM1*—has a shared biological effect with several classes of drugs and thus might be a druggable target.

ADDICTION

Addiction manifests differently in men and women and provides opportunities to better understand basic mechanisms of disrupted sex-specific behavior, said Deena Walker, assistant professor of behavioral neuroscience at Oregon Health & Science University. Men tend to use drugs at a greater rate than women, but women progress to dependence more quickly, report greater craving during withdrawal, are more likely to relapse, and show greater consumption during relapse, putting them at greater risk for overdose, she said (Bobzean et al., 2014). Robust sex differences are also seen in risk of alcohol use disorder, although it is unclear which genetic variants underlie the qualitative difference in risk seen in twin studies or differ in their quantitative effects, said Rohan Palmer, a behavioral geneticist and assistant professor of psychology at Emory University. There is still room for improvement in this area, he said, in part because females account for only about 10 percent of postmortem human brain samples from individuals with overdose-related deaths.

Multiple factors contribute to these sex differences, said Walker. For example, she said neuropharmacological studies indicate that amphetamines induce less release of striatal dopamine in women and that women report less euphoric effects of amphetamines. Adolescent experience and adolescent stress also contribute to sex differences in motivation and reward that influence the risk of addiction, said Walker. Her research as a postdoctoral fellow in Nestler's lab using an adolescent stress paradigm in mice demonstrated that social isolation drives a big sex difference in behavior: In comparison to group-housed animals where males and females showed an equal preference for cocaine, socially isolated males showed a greater preference for cocaine while socially isolated females showed a decreased preference (Walker et al., 2020).[2]

Walker and colleagues examined transcriptional differences in animals displaying sex-specific behavioral responses to cocaine using the social isolation stress model. As was shown earlier in depression and PTSD, in group-housed animals there was little overlap between males and females in terms of the transcriptional response to cocaine. However, there was a gain in the transcriptional response among the socially isolated male animals but not in females, again with little overlap between males and females.

Sexually dimorphic baseline behaviors such as marble burying—males bury more marbles than females—were lost under the stress of social isolation, and these behaviors are also reflected in the transcriptome, said Walker. This observation suggested that the transcriptome might provide information about how behaviors are programmed. To assess changes in global transcriptional structure and potentially identify targets that regulate sex differences in reward, Walker and colleagues used an updated co-expression analytical technique called multiscale embedded gene co-expression network analysis (MEGENA). This technique showed that over the entire transcriptome, socially isolated males gained structure, whereas there was a complete disruption of the structure of the transcriptome in socially isolated females. They also identified one key driver that was conserved across all four groups of mice—*Crym*, the gene for a thyroid hormone–binding protein. They went on to show that by overexpressing *Crym* in the medial amygdala, they could induce a large increase in male-specific cocaine conditioned place preference (CPP), which provides an indirect measure of drug reward, and a decrease in female-specific CPP, thus demonstrating that the medial amygdala is crucial for regulating the sex-specific response to cocaine at both the circuit and the molecular level.

PAIN

Chronic pain is one of the most common comorbidities associated with psychiatric disease, said Theodore (Ted) Price, Eugene McDermott Professor and chair of the Department of Neuroscience in the School of Behavioral and Brain Sciences at The University of Texas at Dallas. Yet, while women and men perceive pain similarly, the underlying mechanisms that cause a transition to chronic pain appear to be quite different, he said. He noted that as with other preclinical research areas, there has been a

---

[2] Made available in preprint format. To learn more, see https://www.biorxiv.org/content/10.1101/2020.02.18.955187v1.full (accessed January 6, 2021).

lag in understanding mechanisms in females because of the historical bias resulting from using only male rodents in studies.

One of the female-specific pain mechanisms being explored in Price's lab involves the calcitonin gene-related peptide (CGRP), which is involved in the pathophysiology of migraine. In addition, new migraine treatments target CGRP or its receptor. Using an inflammatory pain model, Price and colleagues have shown in female mice that a CGRP-sequestering antibody prevented both the development of mechanical hypersensitivity and the transition to a chronic pain state called hyperalgesic priming. In males, the antibody had no such effect, he said. Several anti-CGRP monoclonal antibodies have recently been approved for the treatment of migraine, said Price, although this and other research suggests that for preventing chronic pain, these drugs may be less effective in men than in women (Moehring and Sadler, 2019).

Transcriptomic studies by Price and others have identified many differences in the peripheral immune system that appear to contribute to the transition from acute to chronic pain, known as pain chronification. However, few transcriptomic differences have been seen in nociceptors—the sensory neurons responsible for initiating the pain pathway in the dorsal root ganglion (DRG). Diana Tavares-Ferreira, a postdoctoral fellow in Price's lab, tried an alternative approach to identifying sex differences by assessing the "translatome" of the mouse DRG—the mRNA fragments that are translated into peptides. Using a technique called translating ribosome affinity purification (TRAP), she demonstrated striking sex differences, said Price. Among these is an enzyme called prostaglandin-H2 D-isomerase (PTDGS), which synthesizes the pain mediator prostaglandin D2. Price and colleagues showed that PTDGS and prostaglandin D2 levels are much higher in female mice. Moreover, in this study they showed that male mice injected with PTDGS inhibitors exhibited a robust, dose-dependent pain response, while female mice showed no significant effect, suggesting that baseline prostaglandin D2 levels are protective against pain (Tavares-Ferreira et al., 2020). Price commented that although prostaglandins have long been known to play an important role in pain, the sex difference became apparent only by studying both sexes in preclinical studies.

The Price lab has also been studying pain mechanisms in clinical samples in collaboration with colleagues at the MD Anderson Cancer Center. In well-phenotyped patients with cancer that has infiltrated their vertebrae, doctors at MD Anderson surgically remove DRGs. Price and colleagues then conduct histochemical, electrophysiological, and RNA sequencing studies on DRG neurons from pain and non-pain dermatomes (areas of skin supplied by specific nerves from the DRG). After showing that only the neurons from the pain dermatomes showed spontaneous activity in the nociceptors that drive neuropathic pain, they went on to show striking transcriptomic sex differences, suggesting that different underlying mechanisms may be driving neuropathic pain in males versus females (North et al., 2019). Price suggested that these transcriptomic differences may translate into different therapeutic targets for males and females with neuropathic pain.

Neuropathic pain in males and females also differs at a cellular level, said Price. In males, macrophages are the primary cell type that infiltrates and proliferates in the DRG, whereas in females there is a mix of phenotypically different macrophages, B cells, and possibly T cells, he said. While these different immune cells release different cytokines, the pathways in males and females seem to converge by making nociceptors both spontaneously active and hyperexcitable. This convergence results from the fact that nociceptors express a "dizzying array of receptors," he said. This could explain why antagonists against specific receptors may have limited effectiveness in different population groups, suggested Price.

ADDITIONAL FACTORS CONTRIBUTING TO SEX DIFFERENCES IN STRESS- AND REWARD-RELATED DISORDERS

While the workshop focused on transcriptomic evidence, genetic regulatory networks are also affected by epigenetic mechanisms triggered by environmental influences, including stress, according to Farah Lubin, associate professor of neurobiology at The University of Alabama at Birmingham. Epigenetics, she said, is the study of both heritable and nonheritable regulation of gene expression that occurs without any alteration in the DNA sequence. Neurons appear to have hijacked epigenetic processes such as DNA methylation, posttranslational histone modification, and non-coding RNAs in order to coordinate transcriptional programming across several brain regions, she said. Long non-coding RNAs (lncRNAs) are of particular importance in brain disorders because they appear to play an important role in regulating higher brain functions, said Orna Issler, an instructor at Icahn School of Medicine at Mount Sinai. In depression, at least one-third of the genes that are differentially expressed are lncRNAs, with very little overlap between lncRNAs regulated in males and females, she said.

Exposure to gonadal hormones, may also drive sex differences, said Marianne Seney. Lubin noted that hormone levels change over the life span and may also help to explain the impact of age on disorders.

To conclude the discussion, Eric Nestler mentioned that there are also societal and other non-biological drivers of sex differences. For example, Issler noted that psychosocial factors lead to differences between how boys and girls deal with stress. Nestler added that the stress on parents coping with child care issues during the COVID-19 pandemic also falls disproportionately on women.

3

Transcriptomic Evidence for Sex Differences in Neurodevelopmental and Neurodegenerative Disorders

HIGHLIGHTS

- Striking sex differences in neurodevelopmental and neurodegenerative diseases are reflected in transcriptomic and circuit differences (Gan).
- The higher prevalence of autism spectrum disorders (ASDs) in males may result from differences in biologically-based risk and protective mechanisms (Werling).
- Sex-differential function of glia and/or neurons may contribute to ASD pathobiology or protection (Werling).
- Both genetic and environmental factors may drive the sex differences seen in the onset, symptomatology, and progression of schizophrenia (Roussos).
- In the human brain, differential gene expression among males and females implicates molecular pathways related to epigenome regulation, chromosome X inactivation, hormonal regulation, and synaptic transmission (Roussos).
- The effect size of sex differences in schizophrenia gene expression signatures is small and underscore the challenge of identifying robust sex-by-diagnosis signatures, which will require future analyses in larger cohorts (Roussos).

- Different cell-specific gene expression patterns in male and female brains may contribute to the sex differences seen in Alzheimer's disease prevalence, pathology, and speed of cognitive decline, suggesting that sex should be integrated into precision medicine models of the disease (Hohman).
- Sex differences in how microglia respond to tau may drive the increased prevalence of tauopathies in women (Gan).
- Microglia have also been implicated in schizophrenia, autism, and other brain diseases, suggesting a convergence in the pathophysiological pathways involved (Gan, Stevens).

NOTE: These points were made by the individual speakers identified above; they are not intended to reflect a consensus among workshop participants.

As with the stress-related disorders discussed in Chapter 2, the sex bias for neurodevelopmental and neurodegenerative diseases is striking, said Li Gan, Burton P. and Judith B. Resnick Distinguished Professor of Neurodegenerative Diseases at Weill Cornell Medicine. Advances in transcriptomic and circuit approaches have expanded the understanding of sex biases in these disorders, although much remains to be learned. Nonetheless, recent findings in the study of autism, schizophrenia, Alzheimer's disease (AD), and other tauopathies have provided new opportunities to dissect disease mechanisms, identify new targets, develop biomarkers, and design better preclinical and clinical studies, said Gan.

AUTISM

The pervasive neurodevelopmental disorders known collectively as autism spectrum disorders (ASDs) have about a four-fold higher prevalence in males than in females, although the phenotypic presentation and overall severity are largely similar across both sexes, said Donna Werling, assistant professor of genetics at the University of Wisconsin–Madison (Baio et al., 2018). About 1.7 percent of children in the United States receive an ASD diagnosis on the basis of symptoms in two key domains: social communication deficits and restricted or repetitive behaviors or interests, she said. Many genetic variants have also been associated with increased ASD risk.

One approach to understanding the underlying mechanisms that give rise to these sex differences would be to analyze differences in the molecular status of brain tissue between females and males with autism, said Werling. However, given the fact that phenotypes are similar, a more compelling case could be made for investigating the biology involved in sex-differentiated risk mechanisms. She hypothesized that males may be biologically more vulnerable to certain risk factors and/or that something in the biology of females attenuates the impact of those risk factors such that fewer females present with ASD symptoms (see Figure 3-1). From a transcriptomic perspective, the goal is to find genes and their associated functions that drive male vulnerability and/or female protection.

Werling cited four landmark studies of transcriptomic analysis in brain tissue from people with autism (Gupta et al., 2014; Parikshak et al., 2016; Velmeshev et al., 2019; Voineagu et al., 2011). These studies used non-independent sample sets and, as expected given the difference in prevalence, included more males than females. Thus, said Werling, most of what is known about transcriptomic patterns in the brain comes from only 69 individuals with autism, and only 14 of these are female. These studies also focused on a limited set of brain regions, primarily the frontal and prefrontal cortex and the cerebellum.

The first three of these studies analyzed co-expressed gene modules and showed that in the ASD frontal and temporal cortex there was decreased transcription of modules associated with neuronal and synaptic function and increased expression of modules associated with immune, astrocyte, and

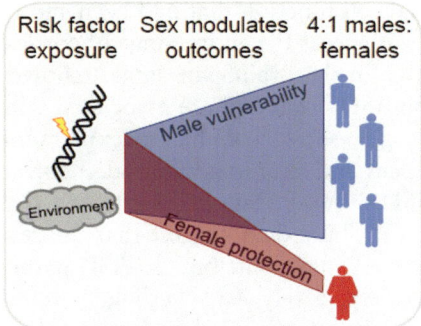
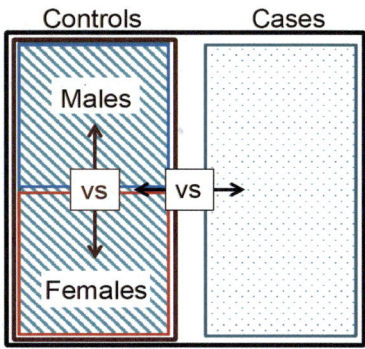

FIGURE 3-1 Characterizing genomic sex differences associated with autism spectrum disorders. The panel on the left illustrates how sex may modulate outcomes in response to risk factor exposure. To assess potential sex-differential risk mechanisms at a transcriptomic level, as shown on the right, a first strategy should characterize the autistic population by comparing males versus females, and evaluate where ASD differences and sex differences intersect.
SOURCE: Presented by Donna Werling, September 23, 2020.

microglial function (Gupta et al., 2014; Parikshak et al., 2016; Voineagu et al., 2011). These patterns were not male specific.

The fourth study sought to understand whether these patterns indicate alterations in cell type composition or function, said Werling. Investigators in Arnold Kriegstein's lab conducted single-cell-expression analysis from the prefrontal cortex and anterior cingulate cortex in 15 donors with ASD (Velmeshev et al., 2019). They identified 17 cell clusters that correspond to specific cortical cell types. Of these, only one cell type was proportionately more abundant in ASD samples than controls—protoplasmic astrocytes. They also conducted differential expression analyses within specific cell types, which showed that many of the most strongly down-regulated genes in cells from patients diagnosed with ASD were primarily in layer two/three excitatory neurons and a class of interneurons called vasoactive intestinal polypeptide interneurons, while the genes that were most strongly up-regulated were observed in protoplasmic astrocytes and microglia.

Taken together, said Werling, these studies show a consistent pattern across tissues and different data modalities of reduced expression of neuronal and synaptic genes and elevated expression of immune and glial genes.

To link these patterns to sex differential risk mechanisms, Werling showed data from an earlier study she conducted as a graduate student in Daniel Geschwind's lab (Werling et al., 2016). Using RNA sequencing data from the BrainSpan consortium,[1] she and her colleagues showed that in the neurotypical cortex, there was female-biased expression of the genes associated with synaptic and neuronal function that had shown reduced expression in brain tissue from people with ASD, and male-biased expression of genes associated with immune and glial cell function that had been shown to be up-regulated in autism. An analysis across the entire range of cortical brain regions and age samples available in the BrainSpan dataset showed that genes that are up-regulated in the ASD brain and are associated with the functions of astrocytes and microglia show male-biased expression, particularly during mid-fetal development and later in adulthood. Neuron-associated genes down-regulated in ASD showed a less striking female bias (Li et al., 2018; Parikshak et al., 2016). These data suggest that the sex-differential function of glia and/or neurons may contribute to ASD pathobiology and/or protective mechanisms, respectively, said Werling.

Although more data are needed to develop a detailed understanding of these sex-related pathobiological and protective mechanisms, transcriptomic studies have provided directions for more focused follow-up, she said. However, these studies have been limited by the relative paucity of brain tissue from autistic females. In addition, she said, to understand the brain circuitry

---

[1] For more information, see https://www.brainspan.org (accessed October 24, 2020).

involved, transcriptomic analysis of more brain regions is needed, as well as data from multiple time points across the life span.

SCHIZOPHRENIA

Schizophrenia is a serious and heterogeneous psychiatric illness with well-established sex differences in incidence, age of onset, symptomatology across the life span, and outcomes, according to Panagiotis Roussos, professor of genetics and genomic sciences and psychiatry at the Icahn School of Medicine at Mount Sinai. For example, onset in men typically occurs in the early 20s, while the incidence in women peaks in the mid- to late 20s and then again in middle age (Abel et al., 2010). Women are more likely to experience depression, while men more often present with negative symptoms such as lack of motivation, anhedonia, and flat affect. Roussos noted that there is conflicting evidence related to sex differences in the expression of positive symptoms such as hallucinations and delusions. As the disease progresses, women are more likely than men to show reduced psychotic symptoms and better cognitive and global functioning, said Roussos. These sex differences suggest that different underlying mechanisms may occur in males and females; furthermore, there is strong evidence for contributions from both genetic and environmental factors, he said.

To examine sex-related transcriptomic changes associated with schizophrenia, Roussos and colleagues turned to the multi-cohort CommonMind Consortium (CMC) dataset,[2] using tissue from four brain banks (Hoffman et al., 2019). This resource enabled them to obtain RNA sequence data on tissue from the dorsolateral prefrontal cortex, Brodmann areas 9 and 46 in 778 individuals (497 males, 281 females). The control to case ratio of 1.3 was consistent between males and females (see Figure 3-2).

Their analysis demonstrated robust and highly reproducible differential gene expression between cases and controls across cohorts, similar to what has been observed in previous studies, said Roussos. For example, the *KCNK1* gene, which codes for a potassium channel subunit, was expressed at lower levels in schizophrenia samples across both the CMC and Human Brain Collection Core (HBCC) cohorts.

Differential expression analysis between males and females also demonstrated concordant sex signatures in the two cohorts. Combined results from the two cohorts identified 686 differentially expressed genes. Not surprisingly, the genes with the biggest effect sizes were located on the X and Y chromosomes, but there were also highly significant sex differences for many more genes residing on autosomes, said Roussos. Pathway analysis on these gene signatures identified molecular pathways related to

---

[2] For more information, see http://commonmind.org (accessed October 26, 2020).

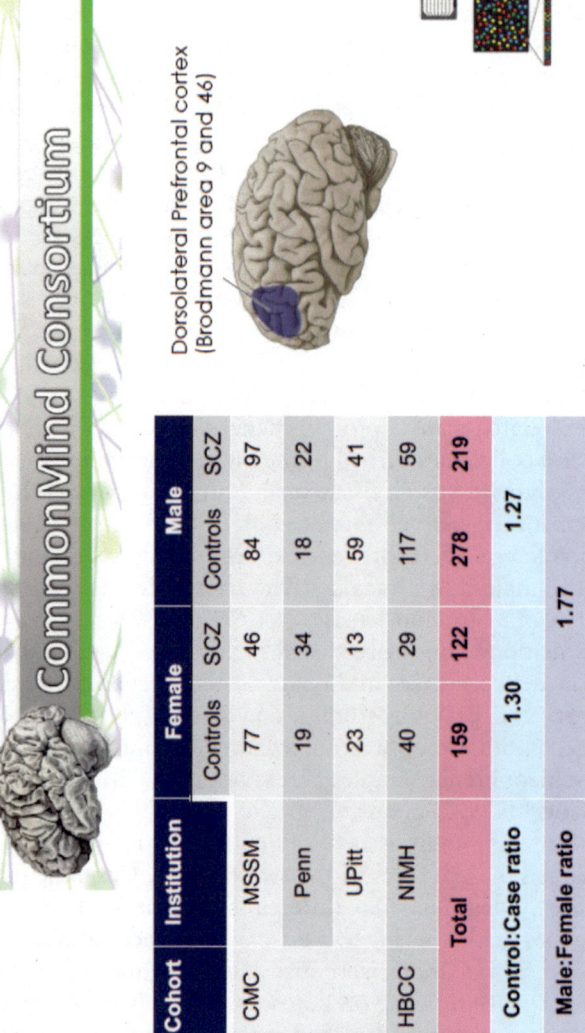

FIGURE 3-2 CommonMind Consortium resources to study gene expression in the human brain.
NOTES: The CommonMind Consortium (CMC) dataset includes the original CMC cohort comprising brains from Mount Sinai, the University of Pennsylvania Brain Bank, and the University of Pittsburgh (the MSSM-Penn-Pitt cohort), as well as the National Institute of Mental Health's Human Brain Collection Core (NIMH-HBCC) cohort, for a total of 778 brains. RNA sequencing studies were conducted on tissue from Brodmann areas 9 and 46.
SOURCE: Presented by Panagiotis Roussos, September 23, 2020.

epigenome regulation, chromosome X inactivation, hormonal regulation, and synaptic transmission.

Next, they performed sex interaction analysis to detect sex-by-diagnosis differences between males and females. Although some genes showed concordance across cohorts, none were significant after multiple test corrections, said Roussos. He suggested that increasing the size of the cohorts would increase the power and could enable identification of significant interactions.

Roussos noted that sex differences in schizophrenia could result either from differences in directionality of gene expression (e.g., genes that are up-regulated in females with schizophrenia, but down-regulated in males with schizophrenia) or from different effect sizes with the same directionality. To examine this possibility, he and his colleagues performed case-control analysis separately for males and females. This analysis indicated that the effect size in females is only 71 percent of that in males, which could explain the more severe clinical phenotype observed in males in other studies.

Roussos and colleagues also used multiscale embedded gene co-expression network analysis (MEGENA) to analyze sex-by-diagnosis differences in co-expression modules rather than individual genes. Many modules yielded robust signals, he said. In a study available in preprint format, pathway analysis indicated that these modules represent molecular functions such as metabolism, hormone synthesis, signaling pathways, and regulation of neurotransmission (Hoffman et al., 2020).

ALZHEIMER'S DISEASE

More than 5 million Americans currently have a diagnosis of AD, and about two-thirds of these are women, said Timothy Hohman, associate professor of neurology at the Vanderbilt University Medical Center (Alzheimer's Association, 2019). Moreover, he said, there is substantial evidence of sex differences in the drivers of AD pathology and the downstream response to pathology, suggesting that sex should be integrated into precision medicine models of the disease.

AD is marked by two primary neuropathologies in the brain—amyloid beta (Aβ) plaques and neurofibrillary tangles composed of tau protein—which drive neurodegeneration and cognitive impairment, said Hohman. Over the past 20 years, therapy development had been driven by the amyloid cascade hypothesis, he said, yet more than 50 clinical trials targeting amyloidosis have failed to result in an effective approved therapy. Hohman presented results from his lab and others integrating sex-specific genomic, transcriptomic, and biomarker data into disease models that aim to identify molecular drivers of AD risk and resilience, which can be translated into novel therapeutic targets.

In both human autopsy studies and mouse models of AD, females have been shown to have higher levels of both Aβ plaques and neurofibrillary tangles, suggesting that the neuropathology is fundamentally different between males and females, said Hohman (Carroll et al., 2010; Oveisgharan et al., 2018; Yue et al., 2011). Moreover, for a given level of neuropathology demonstrated at autopsy, females showed a more rapid decline in cognition compared with males (Barnes et al., 2005). Females also showed more rapid hippocampal atrophy, which is a marker of neurodegeneration, and more rapid cognitive decline in response to AD neuropathology (Koran et al., 2017).

Sex differences have also been demonstrated for genetic risk factors of AD, said Hohman. A large meta-analysis showed that female carriers of the *APOE4* allele, the strongest genetic risk factor for AD, are at higher risk of developing AD than their male counterparts (Neu et al., 2017). Beyond *APOE*, however, Hohman said there are additional sex-specific genomic drivers of AD neuropathology that emerge downstream of amyloidosis, suggesting that there may be a sex-specific genetic architecture of AD. Indeed, there are striking differences in cell-specific gene expression patterns that change in the male and female brain, even in mid-life. For example, with increased age, the male brain shows changes in genes expressed in neurons and genes involved in synaptic transmission and dendritic growth, while the aging female brain shows gene expression changes in many of the support cells of the brain—microglia, endothelial cells, astrocytes, and oligodendrocytes (Sanfilippo et al., 2019). Moreover, this pattern is recapitulated in the AD brain, said Hohman.

Single-cell transcriptomics studies have also demonstrated sex differences in cell types impacted by AD neuropathology, added Hohman. Specifically, neuronal genes are down-regulated in females; while in males, oligodendrocyte genes are up-regulated (Mathys et al., 2019) (see Figure 3-3).

In recent years, sex-specific transcriptomic data have provided many more examples of notable sex differences in transcriptomic networks related to AD, said Hohman. Yet, as with other disease areas, distinguishing cause from consequence remains a major challenge. One approach he and others have used to try to disentangle cause and consequence has been to go back to genome-wide association study (GWAS) data and ask whether genomic predictors act in a sex-specific manner. The original study was a GWAS of cerebrospinal fluid levels of Aβ42, a biomarker of brain amyloid levels. This analysis showed strong associations with several genetic loci—*APOE* on chromosome 19, as well as loci on chromosomes 1 and 6 (Deming et al., 2017). When Hohman and colleagues performed a reanalysis that integrated sex into the model, they showed that the chromosome 6 association was driven entirely by females, and they identified a single-nucleotide

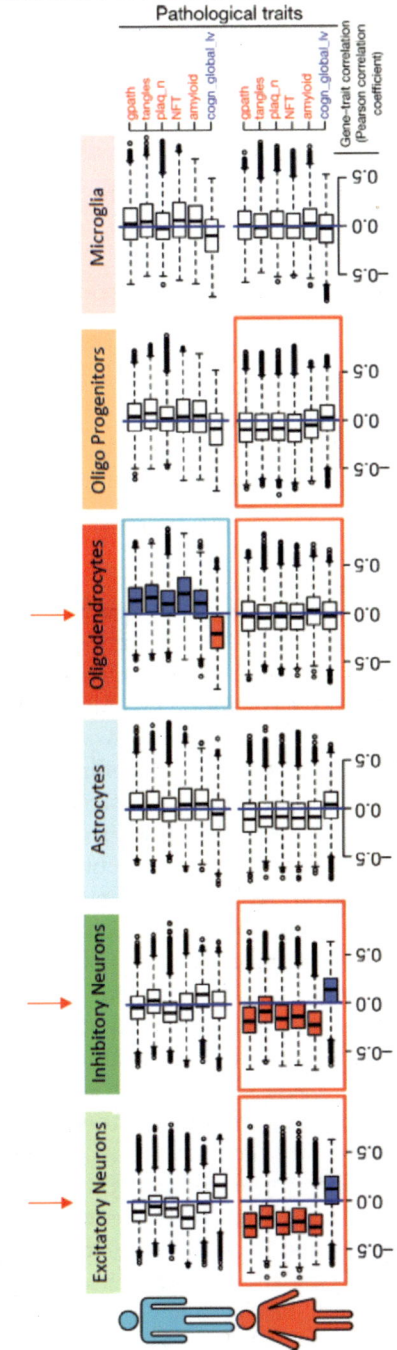

FIGURE 3-3 Sex-specific single-cell transcriptomics in Alzheimer's disease. Gene expression profiles for different cell types differ between men and women. Women (shown in red), but not men (shown in blue), show decreased gene expression in excitatory and inhibitory neurons. Men, but not women, show increased gene expression in oligodendrocytes.
SOURCES: Presented by Timothy Hohman, September 23, 2020; Mathys et al., 2019.

polymorphism responsible for the association that is linked with expression of three different *SERPIN* genes (Deming et al., 2018). *SERPIN*s, according to Hohman, are candidate markers of amyloidosis. They are protease inhibitors that have been shown to inhibit Aβ toxicity, likely by regulating neutrophil infiltration. Interestingly, there are sex differences in the neutrophil infiltration pattern, which appears to be modulated by estradiol. Although the gene is not expressed in the brain, staining for the *SERPINB1* protein in the AD brain reveals its presence all around plaques, said Hohman.

Hohman and colleagues have used the same reanalysis of GWAS data approach to identify sex-specific genomic predictors by looking for associations with positron emission tomography imaging of amyloid, autopsy measures of neurofibrillary tangles, cognitive decline, and resilience to AD. These studies are providing new insight into sex-specific patterns and biological pathways that could be important for understanding how sex interacts with risk of and resilience to AD, he said.

TAUOPATHIES

AD is one of a group of disorders called tauopathies, so named because a pathological hallmark is the deposition of tau protein in the brain as neurofibrillary tangles. AD is not only more common in women, as mentioned earlier, but women also have more tau tangles than men when controlled for *APOE4* carriage and age (Oveisgharan et al., 2018). AD is considered a secondary tauopathy because neurofibrillary tangles coexist with Aβ plaques as well as aberrantly activated microglia surrounding the plaques, added Gan. Long considered a consequence of pathology, she said that microglia are now believed to play a central role, in large part because of recent GWAS data, which have so far identified 29 AD risk loci and potentially 215 genes, many of them enriched in or in some cases exclusively found in microglia and macrophages (Jansen et al., 2019) (see Figure 3-4). Moreover, Gan noted that myeloid cells, such as macrophages and microglia, exhibit the strongest sex differences among immune cells in mice, with greater transcriptomic activation of immune pathways in females (Gal-Oz et al., 2019).

Microglia normally play a protective role as a first responder to injury, clearing aggregates and cell debris and initiating tissue repair through a neurotrophic effect, said Gan. In neurodegenerative disease, microglia respond inappropriately, causing excessive synaptic pruning and release of neurotoxic cytokines and chemokines. To understand sex differences in how microglia respond to tau, Gan and colleagues used RNA sequencing to profile messenger RNA (mRNA) and micro RNA (miRNA) in the brains of P301S transgenic mice, a mouse model of tauopathy (Kodama et al., 2020).

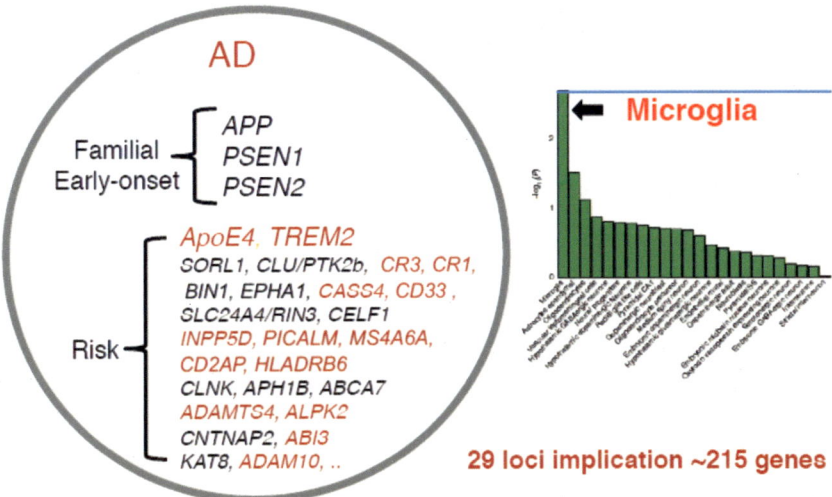

FIGURE 3-4 A meta-analysis identified 29 loci implicated as increasing Alzheimer's disease risk. Those genes highlighted in red are enriched in microglia, as shown in the graph on the right.
SOURCES: Presented by Li Gan, September 23, 2020; Jansen, 2019.

Although the pathological changes are similar in males and females, there was a substantial difference between male and female mice in terms of differential expression of mRNA and miRNA.

To understand the impact on the disease process of differential miRNA expression, they showed that in the absence of Dicer, an enzyme that regulates the maturation and function of miRNA, many more transcripts were modulated in male microglia than in female microglia. When they crossed the Dicer knockouts with tau transgenic mice, they identified a cluster of transcripts in male mice that were nearly absent in female mice. They also showed that ablation of mature miRNAs exacerbated tau pathology in male but not female mice. Taken together, these findings indicate that microglial miRNAs influence homeostasis and tau pathogenesis in a sex-specific manner in tauopathy mice, said Gan.

TREM2 is perhaps the strongest AD risk gene after *APOE* and is highly expressed in microglia, so Gan and colleagues investigated its effects on AD pathology in a sex-specific manner. To do this, they collaborated with Dennis Dickson of the Mayo Clinic, who provided access to a set of brain samples from individuals with a *TREM* mutation called R47H that increases the risk of AD and frontotemporal degeneration (FTD, a primary tauopathy) by 2- to 4.5-fold. By sequencing nearly 85,000 nuclei with either the common variant or R47H, they showed differential expression of microglial genes in males and females with very little overlap. Gan noted that a subcluster of genes that are highly expressed in females but not males were highly enriched for interferon response.

The R47H mutation also exerts strong sex-specific effects on microglial transcriptomes in female but not male mice, said Gan. Female but not male mice with the mutation showed declines in spatial learning and memory.

In addition to their function as mediators of the brain's immune response, microglia also have physiological roles, said Beth Stevens, associate professor of neurology at Harvard Medical School and faculty at the Broad Institute of the Massachusetts Institute of Technology and Harvard. She added that although microglia have been studied in AD and other neurodegenerative diseases, there appears to be a convergence with other brain diseases such as schizophrenia at the level of the biology, genetics, proteomics, and other physiological pathways involved. Single-cell omics and epigenetic studies are "cracking open the field" in exciting ways, and it has become increasingly clear that there are sex differences in various models, especially in the context of environmental perturbations, she said.

For example, as noted earlier, synaptic pruning is an important function of microglia that can lead to pathological synapse loss in AD and other disorders. Several years ago, Steven McCarroll and colleagues identified a structural variant in the complement protein C4 that is the largest common risk factor for schizophrenia (Sekar et al., 2016). More recently, they showed that the same variant also reduces risk for the autoimmune diseases systemic lupus erythematosus and Sjögren's syndrome and that they act more strongly in men than in women (Kamitaki et al., 2020). This observation may provide mechanistic insight into therapeutics and biomarkers for these diseases and offers a molecular foothold with which to dissect mechanisms using induced pluripotent stem cells (IPSCs) as well as nonhuman primate and other animal models, said Stevens.

Because microglia also appear to play a role in autism, Gan suggested that it might be useful to interrogate the pathways involved to determine whether this convergence helps explain sex differences. Werling noted that the two disorders have opposing sex skews in prevalence and that microglia are involved at different stages of development. So there could be completely different processes that just happen to involve the same cell types, or there could be a thread of convergence, she said. Moreover, according to Stevens, making sense of the transcriptomic states of microglia and their relationship to function will require new model systems because their functions are so diverse. She said induced microglial stem cells may help to answer some of these questions by exposing them to different challenges and then assessing single-cell transcriptomics and epigenetics. Other groups are grafting these cells into mouse models with different genetic backgrounds or reporters to see what happens when they get to the brain. Stevens added that access to fresh human brain tissue could also advance understanding of the sex differences in disease-associated microglia (DAM) omics and function. While most of the work on establishing DAM signatures has been done in mouse models, Roussos said his lab has shown that the DAM signature in human brain is very different from that in mouse brain.

Nilüfer Ertekin-Taner, professor of neurology and neuroscience at Mayo Clinic Florida, added that while single-cell analysis can be very informative, analytic approaches that enable deconvoluting existing large-scale, bulk brain RNA-sequencing data could also be useful. She noted that shared datasets from thousands of individuals with a variety of different diseases are available for this type of analysis.

4

Moving Forward

HIGHLIGHTS

- New tools and technologies, including those developed as part of the Brain Research through Advancing Innovative Neurotechnologies (BRAIN) Initiative, have proved useful in understanding sex differences in gene expression and brain circuitry and their impact on disease (Ngai, Stranger).
- The BRAIN Initiative Cell Census Project aims to build an integrated, multi-modal brain atlas as a tool to advance understanding of sex differences in the brain (Ngai).
- Sex differences could have a dramatic impact on how drugs are developed (Zorn).
- To integrate sex differences in drug development, information is needed on mechanistic differences of the compound in men and women, how a drug works differently or has a different safety profile in men and women, and how men and women may use a drug differently (Michelson).
- The National Institutes of Health requires investigators to account for sex as a biological variable in research studies (Clayton).
- The Food and Drug Administration requires new drug applications to present safety and efficacy data by age, race, and gender. It also requires annual reports for investigational new drug data to be presented along these same dimensions (Vasisht).

- Although the number of women enrolled in clinical trials has increased in the past decade, compliance with reporting sex-based differences remains low (Clayton, Laitner).
- Strong evidence has demonstrated sex differences in incidence, risk factors, symptomatology, neuropathology, and biomarkers for neurological diseases (Ertekin-Taner).
- Understanding sex differences in healthy brains can provide insight into disease pathways (Lubin, Seney, Werling).
- To ensure progress in understanding sex differences in brain disorders, sex should be considered at every step of the biomedical research continuum (Clayton, Nestler).
- In addition to studying transcriptomic differences, more research is needed to understand sex differences in the interaction between transcriptomics and genomics, and how those differences drive functional outcomes (Nestler).

NOTE: These points were made by the individual speakers identified above; they are not intended to reflect a consensus among workshop participants.

Understanding sex differences in the brain is one of the major challenges to be addressed as neuroscience moves forward, said Eric Nestler. This will require integrating genomic, transcriptomic, epigenetic, cellular, and circuitry data in order to understand how genome sequence influences function and how it interacts with the environment throughout life, he said. Stevin Zorn, president and chief executive officer of MindImmune Therapeutics, Inc., added that technological innovation alone will not enable achievement of this goal but will need to be coupled with policy changes and consideration of ethical implications (e.g., reducing barriers to clinical trial participation for underrepresented groups).

TECHNOLOGICAL INNOVATION TO DRIVE PROGRESS

Technological innovation has fueled an increased understanding of the underlying genetic and molecular mechanisms that contribute to sex-specific differences in health and disease, said John Ngai, director of the National Institutes of Health's (NIH's) Brain Research through Advancing Innovative Neurotechnologies (BRAIN) Initiative. The BRAIN Initiative was launched in 2014 to develop and apply new tools for understanding how neural circuits underlie complex behaviors. As an example of how new technologies have been applied to the study of sex differences, Ngai pointed to a study by Nirao Shah and colleagues at Stanford University that used bulk RNA profiling to identify a handful of genes that showed sexually dimorphic expression in mouse amygdala and hypothalamus. Interestingly, knocking out these genes affected specific sex-typical behaviors, providing evidence that sex-specific innate behaviors are governed by discrete genetic programs (Xu et al., 2012).

More recently, *Science* published several papers from the NIH Common Fund's Genome-Tissue Expression (GTEx) project, including one focused on the role of sex in gene expression. For example, Barbara Stranger, associate professor of pharmacology at Northwestern University Feinberg School of Medicine, and colleagues showed that about one-third of all genes showed sex differences in expression (Oliva et al., 2020). These differences were subtle and usually restricted to one or two tissues, but in aggregate could have biologically significant effects, said Ngai.

Genes showing sex-specific differences were enriched for a wide spectrum of functions, including drug and hormone responses, epigenetic patterning, embryonic development, tissue morphogenesis, immune response, and cancer, said Stranger. The pattern of sex-differentiated gene expression was highly tissue specific. Stranger said her lab and others have also used expression quantitative trait loci (eQTL) mapping to see if single-nucleotide polymorphisms may have different effects in males versus females. This technique enables identification of genetic loci and candidate genes correlated with traits (Wang et al., 2016). In 44 tissues, they found 366 genes with a sex-biased eQTL signal. These sex-biased eQTLs are present across human tissues and in most cases are driven by a single sex. They could provide clues to understand how sex-biased genetic regulation explains the associations among disease genetics, genes, and mechanisms, said Stranger.

Recognizing that there is much more to learn about sex differences at the genetic and transcriptomic level, Stranger said studies need to be specifically designed to evaluate sex differences in healthy and diseased individuals in longitudinal cohorts across developmental time points, as well as in cell lines.

BRAIN Initiative Cell Census Project

One of the BRAIN Initiative's major coordinated projects, the Cell Census Project, offers opportunities to advance understanding of sex differences in the brain and how they contribute to both health and disease, said Ngai. The concept underlying the project is to build an integrated, multimodal brain cell atlas, he said (see Figure 4-1). Through the use of several advanced single-cell sequencing technologies and spatial transcriptomics techniques, the atlas aims to provide a foundation for obtaining other

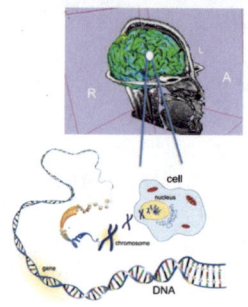
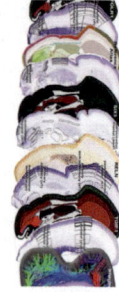

FIGURE 4-1 The BRAIN Initiative Cell Census Project. The Cell Census Project will enable building multiple atlases integrating data on the molecular, anatomical, and functional characteristics of various cell types and the neural circuits that comprise them.
NOTE: ATAC = assay for transposase-accessible chromatin; FISH = fluorescence in situ hybridization; mC = methyl-capture; RNA = ribonucleic acid; seq = sequencing.
SOURCE: Presented by John Ngai, September 23, 2020.

information about the anatomy, morphology, connectivity, and function of cells that constitute neural circuits, said Ngai.

One of the newer technologies that has emerged in recent years—single-cell RNA sequencing—enables investigators to identify the contribution of constituent cell types that constitute a tissue despite their relatively small effect sizes, said Ngai. For example, one of the studies funded by the BRAIN Initiative used this approach to identify genes, neurons, and circuits that contribute to sexually dimorphic neuronal function in the hypothalamic preoptic region (Moffitt et al., 2018). More recently, again with BRAIN Initiative funding, David Anderson and colleagues used deep sequencing single cell profiling to identify 17 transcriptionally distinct cell clusters, several of which were male or female specific (Kim et al., 2019).

Ngai argued that these and other discoveries supported by the BRAIN Initiative lay the foundation for unraveling the molecular and cellular underpinnings of sex-specific behaviors and for identifying sex-specific differences in circuits that are affected in neurological and neuropsychiatric diseases. These discoveries, he said, may guide the development of new, effective, specific, and rational therapies.

ACCOUNTING FOR SEX DIFFERENCES IN THERAPEUTIC DEVELOPMENT

Developing therapies for brain disorders that account for sex differences in disease presentation or response to treatment will be a long process, said Zorn. The challenge in a resource-limited world is to determine when the time is right to invest limited resources so that the data on sex differences can be translated into actions that are based on data-driven hypotheses, he said (IOM, 2011).

The Industry Perspective

In the context of drug development, David Michelson, chief medical officer at Regenacy Pharmaceuticals, said consideration of sex differences must fit into the overall drug development framework, which focuses on pharmacology and predictions about pharmacokinetics, efficacy, and safety. In addition to sex differences, he said, developers must also consider other subpopulations such as children, the elderly, and people with specific comorbidities, among others.

Two categories of information need to be collected, said Michelson. First is understanding how a drug in development works differently in men and women, whether it has a different safety profile, and whether there will be differences between the way men and women will use the drug. The information provided by these studies is limited by the size of the sample and distribution of men and women, he said. He added that the types of studies required may differ depending on the drug and the intended indication, and that some drugs may not require studies on sex-specific differences. If there is empirical support coming out of the laboratory for some sort of sex difference, study designs can be better tailored to either confirm or refute what was predicted, said Michelson.

The second set of studies are more exploratory and tend to be more hypothesis driven as they assess potential sex differences at the mechanistic level, said Michelson. These studies are informed by predictions emerging from preclinical studies, what is known about the mechanism, and what is known about the differential impact of the compound in men and women. Then the developer must determine how much more deeply to study the effects of sex and what essential questions to ask. He noted that the process is challenging given resource limitations. Michelson added that post-approval data may provide additional information that was not uncovered during the core development process.

Melissa Laitner, director of public policy and government affairs at the Society for Women's Health Research, added that patient demographics could help identify who should be included in trials to ensure representation that is proportional to disease prevalence. Laitner also highlighted the barriers to trial participation. For example, she said, women and certain underserved groups face more caregiving, transportation, and financial barriers. Decentralizing clinical trials or adopting digital technologies for data collection could potentially mitigate some of these barriers, said Laitner.

POLICY IMPLICATIONS OF INCORPORATING SEX AS A BIOLOGICAL VARIABLE INTO RESEARCH AND DRUG DEVELOPMENT

In 2014, NIH announced that as part of its efforts to ensure rigor and transparency in taxpayer-funded research, the agency would require investigators to account for sex as a biological variable (SABV) in all funded research, said Janine Clayton, associate director for research on women's health and director of the NIH Office of Research on Women's Health (ORWH) (Clayton, 2016). The policy applies to research designs, analysis, and reporting for vertebrate animal and human studies, and requires scientific justification for single-sex studies. For basic and hypothesis-generating research, it may be sufficient to observe and report sex-based data, she said. However, for preclinical research where the intent is to go to the clinic, the research design itself must incorporate SABV, whether that means employing factorial designs or other strategies. In the clinical space, research designs should lead to increased understanding of the differences in how a disease manifests in men and women; how interventions, diagnostics, or other perturbations affect men and women differently; and what is the clinical meaningfulness of those differences, said Clayton. Finally, sex differences should inform the delivery of care, she added.

The 2016 NIH policy was not the first initiative designed to ensure consideration of sex differences in research. The NIH Revitalization Act of 1993 required NIH-funded clinical trials to include women and minorities as participants and to assess outcomes according to sex, race, and ethnicity (NIH, 1994). Clayton said some progress has been made. NIH data indicate women represent at least 50 percent of NIH-supported clinical research and trials, yet Geller and colleagues (2018) have shown that compliance with sex-specific reporting remains low, she added. As shown in Figure 4-2, only about one-quarter of randomized controlled trials in 2015 analyzed data by sex, and in most of those cases no justification was given for those that did not (Geller et al., 2018). Inadequate reporting means that the return on investment is not being realized for these trials, said Clayton, noting that better SABV reporting would allow other investigators to conduct additional analyses, including meta-analyses of data.

The trans-NIH strategic plan for women's health research, published in 2018, established five goals to advance women's health research

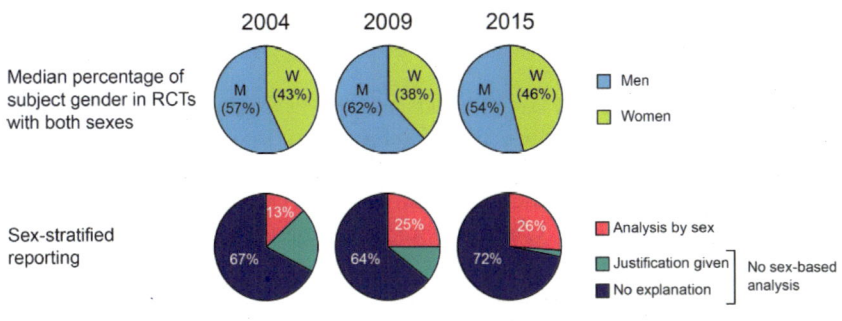

FIGURE 4-2 Sex-specific results reporting in clinical trials. While enrollment of women in randomized controlled trials has increased over time, sex-stratified reporting of data remains low, often with no justification provided.
NOTE: RCT = randomized controlled trial; SABV = sex as a biological variable.
SOURCES: Presented by Janine Clayton, September 23, 2020; adapted from a subset of data presented by Geller et al., 2018.

(NIH, 2018). Clayton provided an overview for three of these goals and described several NIH programs designed to reach the first goal—advancing rigorous research relevant to the health of women, including research on biological differences between females and males, sex differences in health and disease, effects of exposure on disease outcomes, and the mind–body connection as it pertains to sex and gender. These programs include the following:

- Specialized Centers of Research Excellence (SCORE)[1]—Funded through U54 grants, these disease-agnostic centers support basic, clinical, and translational research; provide career development awards for pilot studies often to junior faculty (distinct from the Building Interdisciplinary Research Careers in Women's Health [BIRCWH] program[2]); and support educational opportunities.

---

[1] For more information, see https://orwh.od.nih.gov/womens-health-research/interdisciplinary-research/specialized-centers-research-excellence-sex (accessed November 27, 2020).
[2] For more information, see https://orwh.od.nih.gov/career-development-education/building-interdisciplinary-research-careers-womens-health-bircwh (accessed February 3, 2021).

- First ever trans-NIH R01 (RFA-OD-19-029)—The Intersection of Sex and Gender Influences on Health and Disease, a partnership between ORWH and 11 institutes and centers across NIH.
- Funding for sex and gender administrative supplements, for example, to add subjects or do additional analyses.

The second goal focuses on methods and the leveraging of data sources to examine sex and gender influences. To achieve this goal, ORWH is developing checklists and tools for large-scale analysis of grant applications, and is deploying an inclusion outreach toolkit to engage, recruit, and retain diverse women in clinical studies. Clayton noted that the 21st Century Cures Act reaffirmed NIH's commitment to inclusion across sex, age, race, and ethnicity. The Act also established a task force to increase coordination of research pertaining to pregnant and lactating women, she said. This extends to preclinical research as well, where it is crucial to not only include female animals, but females across the reproductive cycle and life span, added Laitner.

Progress in women's health research can only be achieved through a well-trained, robust, and diverse workforce, which is the focus of the fourth strategic goal, said Clayton. She noted that women are underrepresented in science, technology, engineering, and mathematics (STEM) careers, particularly at higher career levels. Additionally, she said, fewer than 40 percent of medical schools include sex and gender studies in their curricula, and the numbers are even lower for dental and pharmacy schools.

The Food and Drug Administration's (FDA's) Office of Women's Health (OWH) advances a women's health agenda through scientific programs, research funding, training, consultation, and consumer education, said Kaveeta Vasisht, associate commissioner for women's health and director of OWH at FDA. OWH also serves as a principal advisor to the FDA commissioner on scientific, ethical, and policy issues as they pertain to the health of women, she said.

FDA guidance[3] recommends that preclinical studies include animals of both sexes. In 1998, the agency issued a regulation that required new drug applications to present safety and efficacy data by age, race, and gender; another 1998 regulation[4] required annual reports for investigational new drug data to be presented by age, race, and gender. The agency published a Women's Health Research Roadmap in 2015[5] to optimize OWH research

---

[3] For more information, see https://www.fda.gov/media/71542/download (accessed February 3, 2021) and https://www.fda.gov/media/82725/download (accessed February 3, 2021).

[4] For more information, see https://www.fda.gov/science-research/clinical-trials-and-human-subject-protection/investigational-new-drug-applications-and-new-drug-applications-2111998 (accessed February 3, 2021).

[5] For more information, see https://www.fda.gov/science-research/womens-health-research/womens-health-research-roadmap (accessed November 6, 2020).

funding initiatives across FDA and to inform the agency's regulatory work and optimize the health of women, said Vasisht. The roadmap outlined seven priority areas, including advancing safety and efficacy, advancing biomarker science, evaluating new modeling and simulation approaches, and identifying sex differences via emerging technologies, and others.

Vasisht described some of the recent research undertaken by FDA in the area of sex differences. For example, FDA OWH–funded researchers have used exome and RNA sequencing data to evaluate sex differences in Alzheimer's disease and have evaluated transcriptomics- and epigenetics-based predictions of sex- and age-related susceptibilities to treatment-induced adverse effects.

Working in collaboration with NIH ORWH, Vasisht said NIH ORWH and FDA have also created a set of career development educational models, including online courses on integrating sex and gender across the bench to bedside continuum to improve human health.[6] OWH also sponsors a scientific speaker series on topics related to sex and gender differences in health, disease, and response to treatments, she said. The intent of these lectures is to educate staff across FDA's multiple offices and centers and federal partners about the cutting-edge science that advances understanding of sex and gender considerations.

There are several ways to engage and collaborate with FDA, said Vasisht. They can fund research through competitive mechanisms, such as contracts awarded under the FDA Broad Agency Announcement[7] and cooperative agreements with academic institutions, known as Centers of Excellence in Regulatory Science and Innovation.[8] In addition, Cooperative Research and Development Agreements[9] and Memoranda of Understanding,[10] both unfunded, are other ways to collaborate with FDA.

In addition to funding, FDA provides many other opportunities for stakeholders to engage with the agency. FDA's Center for Drug Evalua-

---

[6] For more information, see https://orwh.od.nih.gov/career-development-education/e-learning/bench-bedside (accessed November 6, 2020).

[7] For more information, see https://www.fda.gov/science-research/advancing-regulatory-science/regulatory-science-extramural-research-and-development-projects (accessed November 8, 2020).

[8] For more information, see https://www.fda.gov/science-research/advancing-regulatory-science/centers-excellence-regulatory-science-and-innovation-cersis (accessed November 8, 2020).

[9] For more information, see https://www.fda.gov/science-research/fda-technology-transfer-program/cooperative-research-and-development-agreements-cradas (accessed November 8, 2020).

[10] For more information, see https://www.fda.gov/about-fda/partnerships-enhancing-science-through-collaborations-fda/fda-memoranda-understanding (accessed November 8, 2020).

tion and Research convenes Critical Path Innovation Meetings (CPIMs).[11] CPIM is a forum for FDA and stakeholders to discuss potential scientific advancements in drug development. FDA's Center for Biological Evaluation and Research (CBER) convenes Initial Targeted Engagement for Regulatory Advice on CBER Products meetings[12] to provide informal and non-binding consultation opportunities for sponsors regarding innovative investigational products. A relatively new program at FDA, the Advancing Alternative Methods Working Group,[13] enables stakeholders to engage with regulatory authorities in discussions about novel, innovative technologies and methods, said Vasisht.

Stakeholders also include nonprofit and advocacy groups, such as the Society for Women's Health Research, as well as scientific societies and associations and journal editors and publishers. Laitner highlighted, in particular, the ability of these groups to act as conveners, bringing together interdisciplinary groups of experts to discuss areas of need in women's health research and to strategize about how to move the field forward through collaboration. There is a particular need for stronger policies in the area of therapeutic development, she said, because women are prescribed more drugs than men and report more diverse drug reactions even when data are adjusted for drug dosing issues based on body weight. She cited recent data showing that women are overmedicated and suffer excess side effects because drug dosages are calculated based on studies done overwhelmingly in male subjects (Zucker and Prendergast, 2020). Although FDA regulations passed in 1993 require inclusion of women in drug studies, Laitner noted that many drugs on the market were approved before the regulations were changed. In addition, she noted, many studies still fail to analyze data for sex differences (Woitowich et al., 2020).

Laitner suggested other policy changes that could accelerate research on sex differences, including incorporating sex and gender issues into basic research and design courses; educating grant reviewers, institutional review boards, and institutional animal care review committees about appropriate ways to consider sex and gender in research designs; and overseeing the publication of research findings to ensure that sex and gender are appropriately addressed. In terms of clinical trials and drug approvals, Laitner also suggested better integration of real-world evidence and data on patient experiences.

---

[11] For more information, see https://www.fda.gov/drugs/new-drugs-fda-cders-new-molecular-entities-and-new-therapeutic-biological-products/critical-path-innovation-meetings-cpim (accessed November 8, 2020).

[12] For more information, see https://www.fda.gov/vaccines-blood-biologics/industry-biologics/interact-meetings (accessed November 8, 2020).

[13] To learn more, see https://www.fda.gov/science-research/about-science-research-fda/advancing-alternative-methods-fda (accessed November 8, 2020).

ADDITIONAL AREAS FOR FUTURE RESEARCH

Although the workshop focused on sex differences in various brain disorders, Donna Werling, Marianne Seney, and others noted that a better understanding of sex differences in healthy brains could provide insight into the path to disease. Indeed, said Werling, when comparing males and females, neither one is the prototypical human. Baseline for males and females may be fundamentally different, making it necessary to understand baseline for both sexes at a detailed molecular level, at different stages in development, and in specific brain regions, she said. Farah Lubin added that understanding how gene networks are differentially established and regulated by epigenetic mechanisms in males and females might elucidate commonalities as well as subtle differences that could impact the development of cognitive and other disorders.

Another conundrum facing the field is why syndromes often appear clinically similar and respond to some drugs similarly in men and women even though the underlying biology differs substantially, said Nestler. Seney suggested that drugs might be working on downstream targets that converge across the sexes. Clayton added that some drugs have very broad effects, which could explain common outcomes despite different underlying biology.

A number of therapeutics that appear to affect males and females differently are working their way through the drug development pipeline, and these sex differences could have dramatic impacts on therapeutic development, said Zorn. For example, in the area of neurodegenerative diseases, Nilüfer Ertekin-Taner noted that sex differences have been observed in environmental and genetic factors, transcriptomic changes, biological pathways, comorbidities, and outcomes that include cognition and neuropathology. The evidence for sex differences in incidence, environmental risk factors, symptomatology, neuropathology, and biomarkers is strong, she said, yet there are many knowledge gaps that need to be addressed in the search for new therapies. For example, how do environmental factors affect the epigenome, transcriptome, and disease pathways differently in men versus women; what is the impact of lifelong changes in hormonal status; are there different longitudinal changes in the peripheral transcriptome of men and women and how do they affect disease progression and outcomes; and what sex differences are seen across multiethnic populations?

To understand how these changes occur through a person's lifetime, Ertekin-Taner advocated leveraging peripheral tissue collections and longitudinal cohorts to conduct multi-omics studies, focusing on the transcriptome as well as other omics and integrating other genetic, outcome, and biomarker data. Integrative analyses should also incorporate demographic, socioeconomic, educational, and other lifestyle data, she said. Finally, new model systems are needed to investigate the role of chromosomal sex, hormone influences, and transcriptional and epigenetic changes in brain tissue and cell models.

Nestler emphasized that although the workshop focused on transcriptional differences, further research is also needed on sex differences in the interaction between transcriptomics and genomics. These interactions include translational modifications that are mediated through non-transcriptional mechanisms, cellular and synaptic mechanisms at both the structural and functional levels, and brain circuitry. He suggested that brain circuitry differences between males and females might reflect transcriptomic mechanisms that are modified by the environment from the earliest stages of development through old age.

While there remains an open discussion in the field on areas of future research, other questions also needing to be addressed, said Nestler, include how sex differences may impact functional changes reflected in the genome sequence; interactions between the genome and environment throughout life at transcriptional, translational, post-translational, cellular, synaptic, and circuit levels; and ultimately, how these impact behavior. In addition, it would be crucial to develop resources to gain access to post-mortem human brain tissue of people who do not fall along the male/female binary, for example, transgender individuals, those who have transitioned sex, and intersex individuals, to include in this type of research, he added.

CLOSING THOUGHTS

The workshop clarified and confirmed the fact that the underlying biology of many brain disorders is fundamentally different between men and women, said Nestler. Thus, he said, research programs need to consider sex differences at the earliest stage of planning and study design. Indeed, said Clayton, "until the biomedical research enterprise collectively realizes that this is important enough for us to do in a coordinated manner, we are not going to get the progress that we need." Learning about the effects of sex on response to a therapeutic intervention during phase 3 clinical trials is far too late, she said, advocating instead for sex to be considered in an integrated fashion along the biomedical research continuum at every step, from basic research to marketing approval.

Clayton suggested that convening stakeholders across sectors to reach convergence on how to tackle a problem is essential. Bringing the ecosystem together to think about sex differences in terms of identifying new targets, understanding disease pathogenesis, and designing preclinical and clinical studies is needed, said Zorn, because no one can do this alone.

A

References

Abel, K. M., R. Drake, and J. M. Goldstein. 2010. Sex differences in schizophrenia. *International Review of Psychiatry* (Abingdon, England) 22(5):417–428. https://doi.org/10.31 09/09540261.2010.515205.

Alzheimer's Association. 2019. 2019 Alzheimer's disease facts and figures. *Alzheimer's & Dementia* 15(3):321–387. https://doi.org/10.1016/j.jalz.2019.01.010.

Baio, J., L. Wiggins, D. L. Christensen, M. J. Maenner, J. Daniels, Z. Warren, M. Kurzius-Spencer, L.-C. Lee, S. Pettygrove, C. Robinson, E. Schulz, C. Wells, M. S. Wingate, W. Zahorodny, and M. Yeargin-Allsopp. 2018. Prevalence and characteristics of autism spectrum disorder among children aged 8 years—Autism and Developmental Disabilities Monitoring Network, 11 Sites, United States, 2012. *Morbidity and Mortality Weekly Report Surveillance Summaries* 65(13):1–23. http://dx.doi.org/10.15585/mmwr.ss6513a1.

Barnes, L. L., R. S. Wilson, J. L. Bienias, J. A. Schneider, D. A. Evans, and D. A. Bennett. 2005. Sex differences in the clinical manifestations of Alzheimer disease pathology. *Archives of General Psychiatry* 62(6):685–691. https://doi.org/10.1001/archpsyc.62.6.685.

Blacker, C. J., M. A. Frye, E. Morava, T. Kozicz, and M. Veldic. 2019. A review of epigenetics of PTSD in comorbid psychiatric conditions. *Genes* 10(2):140. https://doi.org/10.3390/genes10020140.

Bobzean, S. A. M., A. K. DeNobrega, and L. I. Perrotti. 2014. Sex differences in the neurobiology of drug addiction. *Experimental Neurology* 259(September):64–74. https://doi.org/10.1016/j.expneurol.2014.01.022.

Carroll, J. C., E. R. Rosario, S. Kreimer, A. Villamagna, E. Gentzschein, F. Z. Stanczyk, and C. J. Pike. 2010. Sex differences in β-amyloid accumulation in 3xTg-AD mice: Role of neonatal sex steroid hormone exposure. *Brain Research* 1366(December):233–245. https://doi.org/10.1016/j.brainres.2010.10.009.

Clayton, J. A.. 2016. Studying both sexes: A guiding principle for biomedicine. *The FASEB Journal* 30(2):519–524. https://doi.org/10.1096/fj.15-279554.

Deming, Y., Z. Li, M. Kapoor, O. Harari, J. L. Del-Aguila, K. Black, D. Carrell, Y. Cai, M. V. Fernandez, J. Budde, S. Ma, B. Saef, B. Howells, K.-L. Huang, S. Bertelsen, A. M. Fagan, D. M. Holtzman, J. C. Morris, S. Kim, A. J. Saykin, P. L. De Jager, M. Albert, A. Moghekar, R. O'Brien, M. Riemenschneider, R. C. Petersen, K. Blennow, H. Zetterberg, L. Minthon, V. M. Van Deerlin, V. M.-Y. Lee, L. M. Shaw, J. Q. Trojanowski, G. Schellenberg, J. L. Haines, R. Mayeux, M. A. Pericak-Vance, L. A. Farrer, E. R. Peskind, G. Li, A. F. Di Narzo, Alzheimer's Disease Neuroimaging Initiative; Alzheimer Disease Genetic Consortium, J. S. K. Kauwe, A. M. Goate, and C. Cruchaga. 2017. Genome-wide association study identifies four novel loci associated with Alzheimer's endophenotypes and disease modifiers. *Acta Neuropathologica* 133(5):839–856. https://doi.org/10.1007/s00401-017-1685-y.

Deming, Y., L. Dumitrescu, L. L. Barnes, M. Thambisetty, B. Kunkle, K. A. Gifford, W. S. Bush, L. B Chibnik, S. Mukherjee, P. L. De Jager, W. Kukull, M. Huentelman, P. K. Crane, S. M. Resnick, C. D. Keene, T. J. Montine, G. D. Schellenberg, J. L. Haines, H. Zetterberg, K. Blennow, E. B. Larson, S. C. Johnson, M. Albert, A. Moghekar, J. L. Del Aguila, M. V. Fernandez, J. Budde, J. Hassenstab, A. M. Fagan, M. Riemenschneider, R. C. Petersen, L. Minthon, M. J Chao, V. M. Van Deerlin, V. M-Y Lee, L. M. Shaw, J. Q. Trojanowski, E. R. Peskind, G. Li, L. K. Davis, J. M. Sealock, N. J. Cox, Alzheimer's Disease Neuroimaging Initiative; Alzheimer Disease Genetics Consortium, A. M. Goate, D. A. Bennett, J. A. Schneider, A. L. Jefferson, C. Cruchaga, and T. J. Hohman. 2018. Sex-specific genetic predictors of Alzheimer's disease biomarkers. *Acta Neuropathologica* 136(6):857–872. https://doi.org/10.1007/s00401-018-1881-4.

Gal-Oz, S. T., B. Maier, H. Yoshida, K. Seddu, N. Elbaz, C. Czysz, O. Zuk, B. E. Stranger, H. Ner-Gaon, and T. Shay. 2019. ImmGen report: Sexual dimorphism in the immune system transcriptome. *Nature Communications* 10(1):4295. https://doi.org/10.1038/s41467-019-12348-6.

Geller, S. E., A. R. Koch, P. Roesch, A. Filut, E. Hallgren, and M. Carnes. 2018. The more things change, the more they stay the same: A study to evaluate compliance with inclusion and assessment of women and minorities in randomized controlled trials. *Academic Medicine: Journal of the Association of American Medical Colleges* 93(4):630–635. https://doi.org/10.1097/ACM.0000000000002027.

Girgenti, M. J., J. Wang, D. Ji, D. Cruz, Traumatic Stress Brain Research Study Group, M. B. Stein, J. Gelernter, K. Young, B. R. Huber, D. E. Williamson, M. J. Friedman, J. H. Krystal, H. Zhao, and R. S. Duman. 2021. Transcriptomic organization of human brain in post-traumatic stress disorder. *Nature Neuroscience* 24:24–33. https://doi.org/10.1038/s41593-020-00748-7.

Gupta, S., S. E. Ellis, F. N. Ashar, A. Moes, J. S. Bader, J. Zhan, A. B. West, and D. E. Arking. 2014. Transcriptome analysis reveals dysregulation of innate immune response genes and neuronal activity-dependent genes in autism. *Nature Communications* 5(December):5748. https://doi.org/10.1038/ncomms6748.

Hoffman, G. E., J. Bendl, G. Voloudakis, K. S. Montgomery, L. Sloofman, Y.- C. Wang, H. R. Shah, M. E. Hauberg, J. S. Johnson, K. Girdhar, L. Song, J. F. Fullard, R. Kramer, C.- G. Hahn, R. Gur, S. Marenco, B. K. Lipska, D. A. Lewis, V. Haroutunian, S. Hemby, P. Sullivan, S. Akbarian, A. Chess, J. D. Buxbaum, G. E. Crawford, E. Domenici, B. Devlin, S. K. Sieberts, M. A. Peters, and P. Roussos. 2019. CommonMind Consortium provides transcriptomic and epigenomic data for schizophrenia and bipolar disorder. *Scientific Data* 6(1):180. https://doi.org/10.1038/s41597-019-0183-6.

Hoffman, G. E., Y. Ma, K. S. Montgomery, J. Bendl, M. Kumar Jaiswal, A. Kozlenkov, CommonMind Consortium, M. A. Peters, S. Dracheva, J. F. Fullard, A. Chess, B. Devlin, S. K. Sieberts, and P. Roussos. 2020. Sex differences in the human brain transcriptome of cases with schizophrenia. Preprint. *Genomics*. https://doi.org/10.1101/2020.10.05.326405.

IOM (Institute of Medicine). 2001. *Exploring the biological contributions to human health: Does sex matter?* Washington, DC: National Academy Press.

IOM. 2011. *Sex differences and implications for translational neuroscience research: Workshop summary.* Washington, DC: The National Academies Press.

Jansen, I. E., J. E. Savage, K. Watanabe, J. Bryois, D. M. Williams, S. Steinberg, J. Sealock, I. K. Karlsson, S. Hägg, L. Athanasiu, N. Voyle, P. Proitsi, A. Witoelar, S. Stringer, D. Aarsland, I. S. Almdahl, F. Andersen, S. Bergh, F. Bettella, S. Bjornsson, A. Braekhus, G. Bråthen, C. de Leeuw, R. S. Desikan, S. Djurovic, L. Dumitrescu, T. Fladby, T. J. Hohman, P. V. Jonsson, S. J. Kiddle, A. Rongve, I. Saltvedt, S. B. Sando, G. Selbaek, M. Shoai, N. G. Skene, J. Snaedal, E. Stordal, I. D. Ulstein, Y. Wang, L. R. White, J. Hardy, J. Hjerling-Leffler, P. F. Sullivan, W. M. van der Flier, R. Dobson, L. K. Davis, H. Stefansson, K. Stefansson, N. L. Pedersen, S. Ripke, O. A. Andreassen, and D. Posthuma. 2019. Genome-wide meta-analysis identifies new loci and functional pathways influencing Alzheimer's disease risk. *Nature Genetics* 51(3):404–413. https://doi.org/10.1038/s41588-018-0311-9.

Kamitaki, N., A. Sekar, R. E. Handsaker, H. de Rivera, K. Tooley, D. L. Morris, K. E. Taylor, C. W. Whelan, P. Tombleson, L. M. Olde Loohuis, Schizophrenia Working Group of the Psychiatric Genomics Consortium, M. Boehnke, R. P. Kimberly, K. M. Kaufman, J. B. Harley, C. D. Langefeld, C. E. Seidman, M. T. Pato, C. N. Pato, R. A. Ophoff, R. R. Graham, L. A. Criswell, T. J. Vyse, and S. A. McCarroll. 2020. Complement genes contribute sex-biased vulnerability in diverse disorders. *Nature* 582(7813):577–581. https://doi.org/10.1038/s41586-020-2277-x.

Kessler, R. C., P. Berglund, O. Demler, R. Jin, D. Koretz, K. R. Merikangas, A. J. Rush, E. E. Walters, P. S. Wang, and National Comorbidity Survey Replication. 2003. The epidemiology of major depressive disorder: Results from the National Comorbidity Survey Replication (NCS-R). *JAMA* 289(23):3095–3105. https://doi.org/10.1001/jama.289.23.3095.

Kim, D.-W., Z. Yao, L. T. Graybuck, T. K. Kim, T. Nghi Nguyen, K. A. Smith, O. Fong, L. Yi, N. Koulena, N. Pierson, S. Shah, L. Lo, A.-H. Poil, Y. Oka, L. Pachter, L. Cai, B. Tasic, H. Zeng, and D. J. Anderson. 2019. Multimodal analysis of cell types in a hypothalamic node controlling social behavior. *Cell* 179(3):713–728. https://doi.org/10.1016/j.cell.2019.09.020.

Kodama, L., E. Guzman, J. I. Etchegaray, Y. Li, F. A. Sayed, L. Zhou, Y. Zhou, L. Zhan, D. Le, J. C. Udeochu, C. D. Clelland, Z. Cheng, G. Yu, Q. Li, K. Kosik, and L. Gan. 2020. Microglial microRNAs mediate sex-specific responses to tau pathology. *Nature Neuroscience* 23(2):167–171. https://doi.org/10.1038/s41593-019-0560-7.

Koran, M. E. I., M. Wagener, T. J. Hohman, and Alzheimer's Neuroimaging Initiative. 2017. Sex differences in the association between AD biomarkers and cognitive decline. *Brain Imaging and Behavior* 11(1):205–213. https://doi.org/10.1007/s11682-016-9523-8.

Labonté, B., O. Engmann, I. Purushothaman, C. Menard, J. Wang, C. Tan, J. R. Scarpa, G. Moy, Y.-H. E. Loh, M. Cahill, Z. S. Lorsch, P. J. Hamilton, E. S. Calipari, G. E. Hodes, O. Issler, H. Kronman, M. Pfau, A. L. J. Obradovic, Y. Dong, R. L. Neve, S. Russo, A. Kasarskis, C. Tamminga, N. Mechawar, G. Turecki, B. Zhang, L. Shen, and E. J. Nestler. 2017. Sex-specific transcriptional signatures in human depression. *Nature Medicine* 23(9):1102–1111. https://doi.org/10.1038/nm.4386.

Li, M., G. Santpere, Y. Imamura Kawasawa, O. V. Evgrafov, F. O. Gulden, S. Pochareddy, S. M. Sunkin, Z. Li, Y. Shin, Y. Zhu, A. M. M. Sousa, D. M. Werling, R. R. Kitchen, H. J. Kang, M. Pletikos, J. Choi, S. Muchnik, X. Xu, D. Wang, B. Lorente-Galdos, S. Liu, P. Giusti-Rodríguez, H. Won, C. A. de Leeuw, A. F. Pardiñas, BrainSpan Consortium, PsychENCODE Consortium, PsychENCODE Developmental Subgroup, M. Hu, F. Jin, Y. Li, M. J. Owen, M. C. O'Donovan, J. T. R. Walters, D. Posthuma, M. A. Reimers, P.

Levitt, D. R. Weinberger, T. M. Hyde, J. E. Kleinman, D. H. Geschwind, M. J. Hawrylycz, M. W. State, S. J. Sanders, P. F. Sullivan, M. B. Gerstein, E. S. Lein, J. A. Knowles, and N. Sestan. 2018. Integrative functional genomic analysis of human brain development and neuropsychiatric risks. *Science* 362(6420):eaat7615. doi: 10.1126/science.aat7615.

Mathys, H., J. Davila-Velderrain, Z. Peng, F. Gao, S. Mohammadi, J. Z. Young, M. Menon, L. He, F. Abdurrob, X. Jiang, A. J. Martorell, R. M. Ransohoff, B. P. Hafler, D. A. Bennett, M. Kellis, and L.-H. Tsai. 2019. Single-cell transcriptomic analysis of Alzheimer's disease. *Nature* 570(7761):332–337. https://doi.org/10.1038/s41586-019-1195-2.

Moehring, F., and K. E. Sadler. 2019. Female-specific effects of CGRP suggest limited efficacy of new migraine treatments in males. *The Journal of Neuroscience* 39(46):9062–9064. https://doi.org/10.1523/JNEUROSCI.1254-19.2019.

Moffitt, J. R., D. Bambah-Mukku, S. W. Eichhorn, E. Vaughn, K. Shekhar, J. D. Perez, N. D. Rubinstein, J. Hao, A. Regev, C. Dulac, and X. Zhuang. 2018. Molecular, spatial, and functional single-cell profiling of the hypothalamic preoptic region. *Science* 362(6416). https://doi.org/10.1126/science.aau5324.

Nees, F., S. H. Witt, and H. Flor. 2018. Neurogenetic approaches to stress and fear in humans as pathophysiological mechanisms for posttraumatic stress disorder. *Biological Psychiatry* 83(10):810–820. https://doi.org/10.1016/j.biopsych.2017.12.015.

Neu, S. C., J. Pa, W. Kukull, D. Beekly, A. Kuzma, P. Gangadharan, L.-S. Wang, K. Romero, S. P. Arneric, A. Redolfi, D. Orlandi, G. B. Fisoni, R. Au, S. Devine, S. Auerbach, A. Espinosa, M. Boada, A. Ruiz, S. C. Johnson, R. Koscik, J.-J. Wang, W.-C. Hsu, Y.-L. Chen, and A. W. Toga. 2017. Apolipoprotein E genotype and sex risk factors for Alzheimer disease: A meta-analysis. *JAMA Neurology* 74(10):1178–1189. https://doi.org/10.1001/jamaneurol.2017.2188.

Nievergelt, C. M., A. X. Maihofer, T. Klengel, E. G. Atkinson, C.-Y. Chen, K. W. Choi, J. R. I. Coleman, S. Dalvie, L. E. Duncan, J. Gelernter, D. F. Levey, M. W. Logue, R. Polimanti, A. C. Provost, A. Ratanatharathorn, M. B. Stein, K. Torres, A. E. Aiello, L. M. Almli, A. B. Amstadter, S. B. Andersen, O. A. Andreassen, P. A. Arbisi, A. E. Ashley-Koch, S. Bryn Austin, E. Avdibegovic, D. Babić, M. Baevad-Hansen, D. G. Baker, J. C. Beckham, L. J. Bierut, J. I. Bisson, M. P. Boks, E. A. Bolger, A. D. Børglum, B. Bradley, M. Brashear, G. Breen, R. A. Bryant, A. C. Bustamante, J. Bybjerg-Grauholm, J. R. Calabrese, J. M. Caldas-de-Almeida, A. M. Dale, M. J. Daly, N. P. Daskalakis, J. Deckert, D. L. Delahanty, M. F. Dennis, S. G. Disner, K. Domschke, A. Dzubur-Kulenovic, C. R. Erbes, A. Evans, L. A. Farrer, N. C. Feeny, J. D. Flory, D. Forbes, C. E. Franz, S. Galea, M. E. Garrett, B. Gelaye, E. Geuze, C. Gillespie, A. Goci Uka, S. D. Gordon, G. Guffanti, R. Hammamieh, S. Harnal, M. A. Hauser, A. C. Heath, S. M. J. Hemmings, D. M. Hougaard, M. Jakovljevic, M. Jett, E. Otto Johnson, I. Jones, T. Jovanovic, X.-J. Qin, A. G. Junglen, K.-I. Karstoft, M. L. Kaufman, R. C. Kessler, A. Khan, N. A. Kimbrel, A. P. King, N. Koen, H. R. Kranzler, W. S. Kremen, B. R. Lawford, L. A. M. Lebois, C. E. Lewis, S. D. Linnstaedt, A. Lori, B. Lugonja, J. J. Luykx, M. J. Lyons, J. Maples-Keller, C. Marmar, A. R. Martin, N. G. Martin, D. Maurer, M. R. Mavissakalian, A. McFarlane, R. E. McGlinchey, K. A. McLaughlin, S. A. McLean, S. McLeay, D. Mehta, W. P. Milberg, M. W. Miller, R. A. Morey, C. P. Morris, O. Mors, P. B. Mortensen, B. M. Neale, E. C. Nelson, M. Nordentoft, S. B. Norman, M. O'Donnell, H. K. Orcutt, M. S. Panizzon, E. S. Peters, A. L. Peterson, M. Peverill, R. H. Pietrzak, M. A. Polusny, J. P. Rice, S. Ripke, V. B. Risbrough, A. L. Roberts, A. O. Rothbaum, B. O. Rothbaum, P. Roy-Byrne, K. Ruggiero, A. Rung, B. P. F. Rutten, N. L. Saccone, S. E. Sanchez, D. Schijven, S. Seedat, A. V. Seligowski, J. S. Seng, C. M. Sheerin, D. Silove, A. K. Smith, J. W. Smoller, S. R. Sponheim, D. J. Stein, J. S. Stevens, J. A. Sumner, M. H. Teicher, W. K. Thompson, E. Trapido, M. Uddin, R. J. Ursano, L. Luella van den Heuvel, M. Van Hooff, E. Vermetten, C. H. Vinkers, J. Voisey, Y. Wang, Z. Wang, T. Werge, M. A Williams, D. E. Williamson,

S. Winternitz, C. Wolf, E. J. Wolf, J. D. Wolff, R. Yehuda, R. McD. Young, K. A. Young, H. Zhao, L. A. Zoellner, I. Liberzon, K. J. Ressler, M. Haas, and K. C. Koenen. 2019. International meta-analysis of PTSD genome-wide association studies identifies sex- and ancestry-specific genetic risk loci. *Nature Communications* 10(1):4558. https://doi.org/10.1038/s41467-019-12576-w.

NIH (National Institutes of Health). 1994. NIH Guidelines on the inclusion of women and minorities as subjects in clinical research. *Federal Registry* 59:14508–14513.

NIH. 2018. *Advancing science for the health of women: The trans-NIH strategic plan for women's health reasearch—2019-2023.* https://orwh.od.nih.gov/sites/orwh/files/docs/ORWH_Strategic_Plan_2019_02_21_19_V2_508C.pdf (accessed December 15, 2020).

North, R. Y., Y. Li, P. Ray, L. D. Rhines, C. Esteves Tatsui, G. Rao, C. A. Johansson, H. Zhang, Y. H. Kim, B. Zhang, G. Dussor, T. H. Kim, T. J. Price, and P. M. Dougherty. 2019. Electrophysiological and transcriptomic correlates of neuropathic pain in human dorsal root ganglion neurons. *Brain: A Journal of Neurology* 142(5):1215–1226. https://doi.org/10.1093/brain/awz063.

Oliva, M., M. Muñoz-Aguirre, S. Kim-Hellmuth, V. Wucher, A. D. H. Gewirtz, D. J. Cotter, P. Parsana, S. Kasela, B. Balliu, A. Viñuela, S. E. Castel, P. Mohammadi, F. Aguet, Y. Zou, E. A. Khramtsova, A. D. Skol, D. Garrido-Martin, F. Reverter, A. Brown, P. Evans, E. R. Gamazon, A. Payne, R. Bonazzola, A. N. Barbeira, A. R. Hamel, A. Martinez-Perez, J. Manuel Soria, GTEx Consortium, B. L. Pierce, M. Stephens, E. Eskin, E. T. Dermitzakis, A. V. Sergè, H. Kyung Im, B. E. Engelhardt, K. G. Ardlie, S. B. Montgomery, A. J. Battle, T. Lappalainen, R. Guigó, and B. E. Stranger. 2020. The impact of sex on gene expression across human tissues. *Science* 369(6509). https://doi.org/10.1126/science.aba3066.

Oveisgharan, S., Z. Arvanitakis, L. Yu, J. Farfel, J. A. Schneider, and D. A. Bennett. 2018. Sex differences in Alzheimer's disease and common neuropathologies of aging. *Acta Neuropathologica* 136(6):887–900. https://doi.org/10.1007/s00401-018-1920-1.

Parikshak, N. N., V. Swarup, T. G. Belgard, M. Irimia, G. Ramaswami, M. J. Gandal, C. Hartl, V. Leppa, L. de la Torre Ubieta, J. Huang, J. K. Lowe, B. J. Blencowe, S. Horvath, and D. H. Geschwind. 2016. Genome-wide changes in LncRNA, splicing, and regional gene expression patterns in autism. *Nature* 540(7633):423–427. https://doi.org/10.1038/nature20612.

Sanfilippo, C., P. Castrogiovanni, R. Imbesi, D. Tibullo, G. Li Volti, I. Barbagallo, N. Vicario, G. Musumeci, and M. Di Rosa. 2019. Middle-aged healthy women and Alzheimer's disease patients present an overlapping of brain cell transcriptional profile. *Neuroscience* 406(May):333–344. https://doi.org/10.1016/j.neuroscience.2019.03.008.

Sekar, A., A. R. Bialas, H. de Rivera, A. Davis, T. R. Hammond, N. Kamitaki, K. Tooley, J. Presumey, M. Baum, V. Van Doren, G. Genovese, S. A. Rose, R. E. Handsaker, Schizophrenia Working Group of the Psychiatric Genomics Consortium, M. J. Daly, M. C. Carroll, B. Stevens, and S. A. McCarroll. 2016. Schizophrenia risk from complex variation of complement component 4. *Nature* 530(7589):177–183. https://doi.org/10.1038/nature16549.

Seney, M. L., Z. Huo, K. Cahill, L. French, R. Puralewski, J. Zhang, R. W. Logan, G. Tseng, D. A. Lewis, and E. Sibille. 2018. Opposite molecular signatures of depression in men and women. *Biological Psychiatry* 84(1):18–27. https://doi.org/10.1016/j.biopsych.2018.01.017.

Tavares-Ferreira, D., P. R. Ray, I. Sankaranarayanan, G. L. Mejia, A. Wangzhou, S. Shiers, R. Uttarkar, S. Megat, P. Barragan-Iglesias, G. Dussor, A. N. Akopian, and T. J. Price. 2020. Sex differences in nociceptor translatomes contribute to divergent prostaglandin signaling in male and female mice. *Biological Psychiatry* S0006-3223(20):31952-1. doi: 10.1016/j.biopsych.2020.09.022.

Velmeshev, D., L. Schirmer, D. Jung, M. Haeussler, Y. Perez, S. Mayer, A. Bhaduri, N. Goyal, D. H. Rowitch, and A. R. Kriegstein. 2019. Single-cell genomics identifies cell type-specific molecular changes in autism. *Science* 364(6441):685–689. https://doi.org/10.1126/science.aav8130.

Voineagu, I., X. Wang, P. Johnston, J. K. Lowe, Y. Tian, S. Horvath, J. Mill, R. M. Cantor, B. J. Blencowe, and D. H. Geschwind. 2011. Transcriptomic analysis of autistic brain reveals convergent molecular pathology. *Nature* 474(7351):380–384. https://doi.org/10.1038/nature10110.

Walker, D. M., X. Zhou, A. Ramakrishnan, H. M. Cates, A. M. Cunningham, C. J. Peña, R. C. Bagot, O. Issler, Y. Van der Zee, A. P. Lipschultz, A. Godino, C. J. Browne, G. E. Hodes, E. M. Parise, A. Torres-Berrio, P. J. Kennedy, L. Shen, B. Zhang, and E. J. Nestler. 2020. Adolescent social isolation reprograms the medial amygdala: Transcriptome and sex differences in reward. Preprint. *Neuroscience*. https://doi.org/10.1101/2020.02.18.955187.

Wang, Y., R. Richard, and Y. Pan. 2016. Prior knowledge guided EQTL mapping for identifying candidate genes. *BMC Bioinformatics* 17(1):531. https://doi.org/10.1186/s12859-016-1387-9.

Werling, D. M., N. N. Parikshak, and D. H. Geschwind. 2016. Gene expression in human brain implicates sexually dimorphic pathways in autism spectrum disorders. *Nature Communications* 7(February):10717. https://doi.org/10.1038/ncomms10717.

Woitowich, N. C., A. Beery, and T. Woodruff. 2020. A 10-year follow-up study of sex inclusion in the biological sciences. *ELife* 9. https://doi.org/10.7554/eLife.56344.

Xu, X., J. K. Coats, C. F. Yang, A. Wang, O. M. Ahmed, M. Alvarado, T. Izumi, and N. M. Shah. 2012. Modular genetic control of sexually dimorphic behaviors. *Cell* 148(3):596–607. https://doi.org/10.1016/j.cell.2011.12.018.

Yue, M., A. Hanna, J. Wilson, H. Roder, and C. Janus. 2011. Sex difference in pathology and memory decline in RTg4510 mouse model of tauopathy. *Neurobiology of Aging* 32(4):590–603. https://doi.org/10.1016/j.neurobiolaging.2009.04.006.

Zucker, I., and B. J. Prendergast. 2020. Sex differences in pharmacokinetics predict adverse drug reactions in women. *Biology of Sex Differences* 11(June). https://doi.org/10.1186/s13293-020-00308-5.

B

Workshop Agenda

Sex Differences in Brain Disorders:
Emerging Transcriptomic Evidence and Implications for
Therapeutic Development—A Virtual Workshop

September 23, 2020

Virtual via Zoom

Workshop Objectives: This public workshop will bring together experts and key stakeholders from academia, government, industry, and non-profit organizations to explore emerging evidence regarding differences in transcriptomic abnormalities that occur in the brains of men versus women with a variety of brain disorders, including depression, posttraumatic stress disorder, drug addiction, neurodegenerative conditions, and others.

Invited presentations and discussions will be designed to:

- Review the landscape of emerging evidence regarding sex differences in transcriptomic abnormalities in a variety of brain disorders, and discuss how this can be used to advance understanding of brain disorder pathophysiology.
- Explore ramifications for therapeutic development for these disorders, including identification of new targets, implications for preclinical and clinical study design, regulatory considerations, and potential sex-specific treatments.

- Discuss open research questions and opportunities to move the field forward.

10:00am   Welcome and Overview of Workshop
               ERIC NESTLER, Icahn School of Medicine at Mount Sinai, *Workshop Chair*

SESSION I: CURRENT LANDSCAPE OF EMERGING TRANSCRIPTOMIC EVIDENCE FOR SEX DIFFERENCES IN BRAIN DISORDERS

Objectives:
- Provide an overview of the current landscape of emerging evidence regarding sex differences in transcriptomic abnormalities in a variety of brain disorders.
- Consider how this evidence can be used to advance understanding of brain disorder pathophysiology.

10:15am   Session Overview
               RITA VALENTINO, National Institute on Drug Abuse, *Session Co-Moderator*

Part A: Stress- and Reward-Related Disorders

10:20am   Depression
               MARIANNE SENEY, University of Pittsburgh

10:35am   Posttraumatic Stress Disorder
               MATTHEW GIRGENTI, Yale School of Medicine

10:50am   Addiction
               DEENA WALKER, Oregon Health & Science University

11:05am   Pain
               THEODORE PRICE, The University of Texas at Dallas

11:20am   Panel Discussion:
               The speakers above will be joined by panelists:
               FARAH LUBIN, The University of Alabama at Birmingham
               ORNA ISSLER, Icahn School of Medicine at Mount Sinai
               ROHAN PALMER, Emory University

11:40am   General Discussion

12:00pm   Lunch Break
          Attendees will reconvene at 12:40pm for the following lunchtime talk and discussion.

          BRAIN Initiative Cell Census Network—Applications to Understanding Sex Differences
          JOHN NGAI, National Institutes of Health

Part B: Neurodevelopmental and Neurodegenerative Disorders

1:00pm   Panel Overview
          LI GAN, Weill Cornell Medical College,
          Session Co-Moderator

1:05pm   Autism
          DONNA WERLING, University of Wisconsin–Madison

1:20pm   Schizophrenia
          PANAGIOTIS ROUSSOS, Icahn School of Medicine at Mount Sinai

1:35pm   Alzheimer's Disease
          TIMOTHY HOHMAN, Vanderbilt University

1:50pm   Tauopathies
          LI GAN, Weill Cornell Medical College

2:05pm   Panel Discussion
          The speakers above will be joined by panelists:
          BARBARA STRANGER, Northwestern University Feinberg School of Medicine
          BETH STEVENS, Harvard University
          NILÜFER ERTEKIN-TANER, Mayo Clinic

2:25pm   General Discussion

2:45pm   BREAK

SESSION II: MOVING FORWARD—
THERAPEUTIC DEVELOPMENT AND POLICY IMPLICATIONS

Objectives:
- Explore ramifications for therapeutic development for brain disorders, including identification of new targets, implications for preclinical and clinical study design, regulatory considerations, and potential sex-specific treatments.
- Discuss open research questions and opportunities to move the field forward.

3:00pm   Session Overview
          STEVIN ZORN, MindImmune Therapeutics, Inc.,
          Session Moderator

3:05pm   Speakers
          JANINE CLAYTON, National Institutes of Health
          KAVEETA VASISHT, Food and Drug Administration
          DAVID MICHELSON, Regenacy Pharmaceuticals
          MELISSA LAITNER, Society for Women's Health Research

3:55pm   Panel Discussion

4:15pm   General Discussion

4:35pm   Synthesis of Key Workshop Themes and Future Directions
          ERIC NESTLER, Icahn School of Medicine at Mount Sinai,
          Workshop Chair

5:00pm   ADJOURN WORKSHOP